Good
health

ON THE GO!

Good health

ON THE GO!

Anna Niec-Oszywa

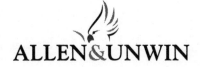

ALLEN&UNWIN

First published in 2001

Allen & Unwin
83 Alexander Street
Crows Nest NSW 2065
Australia
Phone: (61 2) 8425 0100
Fax: (61 2) 9906 2218
Email: info@allenandunwin.com
Web: www.allenandunwin.com

National Library of Australia
Cataloguing-in-Publication entry:

Niec-Oszywa, Anna.
    Good health on the go!

    Bibliography.
    Includes index.
    ISBN 1 86508 509 X.

    1. Nutrition. 2. Diet. 3. Health.
    I. Title.

613.2

Text design by Simon Paterson
Set in 11/15 pt Garamond by Bookhouse
Printed by Griffin Press, Adelaide

10 9 8 7 6 5 4 3 2 1

Note: The nutritional advice
in this book is not intended
to replace the services of a
trained health professional.
Any application of the
suggestions in this book are
at the reader's discretion.

For my husband Gregory

Contents

Introduction   x

part one   Introduction to nutrition

1   The A to Z of nutrition   3
Macronutrients • Micronutrients • The best food sources of
vitamins and minerals • Bioavailability

2   Nutritional variety   19
Working out your food variety score • Using colour as a measure
of food variety • Using models to illustrate optimum nutritional
variety

3   Nutritional supplements   29
Preventing or correcting nutrient deficiencies • Reducing the risk
of chronic conditions • Safety concerns and safety margins

part two   Prevention is better than cure

4   Keeping fit   39
Food—our source of energy • Energy balance • People's energy
needs differ • Estimating your energy needs • Fuel of choice for
exercise • The benefits of exercise • The waist-to-hip ratio—the
shape as well as weight

5 Nutrition and heart health   **65**

Atherosclerosis • Understanding heart disease • Blood cholesterol • Optimum nutrition for heart health • Fat • Essential fats • Antioxidants • Coffee

6 Tuning your immune system   **94**

The role of nutrition in immunity • Antioxidant defences • Free radical quenchers • Trace elements • Compounds with antioxidant properties • Solutions to the antioxidant shortage • Practical manoeuvres in the kitchen • Speedy antioxidant boosters

7 Stress and nutrition   **108**

Diet and stress • Fundamentals of survival: the fight or flight response • Dietary means to counteract the effects of chronic stress • Dietary components that imitate stress reactions • Rigid dieting

8 Nutrition and brain performance   **120**

Food and brain chemistry • Meal composition • Meal times • Reactive hypoglycaemia • The glycaemic index of foods • Overcoming sleep problems • Improve your memory with choline

Conclusion: Looking after your nutrition needs   **136**

Appendix: Eating out   *140*

The art of choosing nutritious meals from the menu • Dining out international style • Aeroplane food

Further reading   *170*

Conversions   *172*

Index   *173*

Health isn't everything,

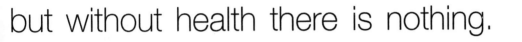

but without health there is nothing.

Introduction

Two seemingly very different gadgets have made the billion-dollar 'slimming' industry what it is today. The computer and the food processor have added many centimetres to many waists: the food processor by tampering with wholesome foods and adding excess energy in the form of sugar and fat; and the computer by creating a work environment that requires us to expend little energy. The end result is obesity, with excess weight a symptom of poor nutrition.

Research shows that adequate nutrition can achieve weight loss, improve fitness and increase your energy levels. It will also improve immunity, may help you to cope better with stress and can improve your cognitive function. It can make a difference between suffering from a debilitating heart disease in your forties or enjoying life to a ripe old age.

This book is based on that scientific research. It is a tool designed to teach you how to achieve optimum nutrition. In each chapter I will guide you through a set of goals and the benefits of achieving those goals. I will then take you through the science behind the scenes, explaining why it is important to make specific changes to your eating habits. We then look at how to put the science into practice.

Checkpoints throughout the book enable you to check your current eating habits—are they up to scratch? You will find out how your diet stands up to the test. Work through the checkpoints, make notes, set your goals and put your nutritional know-how into practice.

Good Health

The manual is designed as a fast learning tool with many practical applications. The appendix covers eating out; it is a guide to the art of choosing nutritious meals in restaurants specialising in different cuisines. Selecting a nutritious, flavoursome meal from any type of menu will soon become second nature to you. All meals are listed first by their original name (to aid in food selection when travelling overseas), followed by their name in English.

The book is intended to offer you the means to fine-tune your eating habits in a fast, efficient way, making changes that will fit into your lifestyle and become permanent.

Enjoy life, enjoy good health!

Anna Niec-Oszywa

part one

Introduction to nutrition

chapter one

The A to Z of nutrition

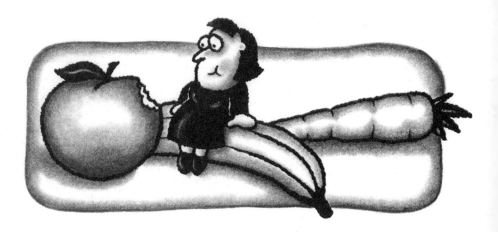

■ GOALS

- To understand the basics of nutrition
- To increase awareness of the sources of different nutrients

■ BENEFITS

- You will be able to distinguish nutritional facts from fallacies
- You will be less likely to suffer from a nutritional imbalance

Nutrition is the science of nourishing the body. Good nutrition prevents the onset of degenerative diseases. It helps to keep our body in good shape for as long as possible. It can add quality years to our life while preserving good health.

Balanced nutrition is a very positive concept, while *dieting* is not. Taking extreme measures to lose weight sacrifices good nutrition. Unsound weight-loss diets have sprouted in our society like mushrooms after rain. It's very important to guide against tunnel vision where weight loss becomes the ultimate goal, more important even than physical and emotional well-being. Most dietary regimes are far removed from balanced nutrition and the concept of health, and so I thoroughly discourage you from following such regimes.

I invite you instead to think about nutrition as a means of optimising your physical and psychological well-being without making radical and unhealthy sacrifices. In order to do so, it's important to develop an understanding of nutritional balance and variety and to exercise your knowledge on a daily basis. Maintaining a balanced diet can be likened to keeping to a sound budget, where the overall aim is to save money in order to better your lifestyle in the future yet still have enough freedom to enjoy the now!

In order to understand what the experts are saying and be able to distinguish the gimmicks from sound scientific advice, you need to master some basic nutritional jargon. Let's start with the terms *macronutrients* and *micronutrients*.

Macronutrients

Macro means present in large quantities, and *nutrients* means food for the body. Thus, *macronutrients* describes carbohydrates, fats, proteins, fibre and fluid. We'll look at each of these in turn.

CARBOHYDRATES

The term *carbohydrate* describes starches and sugars. Starches are called complex carbohydrates, and sugars are called simple carbohydrates. Foods that are rich in complex carbohydrates include pasta, rice, breads, cereals, potato, corn, legumes and fruit. Foods containing simple carbohydrates also include fruit as well as honey, sweet syrups and sweets. When digested, complex carbohydrates, or starches, break down into simple carbohydrates, or sugar. The sugar is called glucose and it's an instant energy source for the body. The main function of carbohydrates in our body is to provide a source of readily available energy.

FATS

Fats are the main source of energy in the diet. On a per weight basis, fats provide the body with more energy than carbohydrates. Fats offer a stand-by source of energy or, if you like, a reserve of energy to be tapped into when our body has run out of glucose stored in the liver and muscles. In addition, fats are the transport vehicles for fat-soluble vitamins.

Two types of fats—linoleic acid and alpha ($\propto$) linolenic acid—can't be made by the body and must be obtained from the diet. These are called essential fatty acids. Good sources of essential fatty acids are nuts, seeds and vegetables. We will look at these fats in more detail in Chapter 5.

For more information on the fat content of foods, visit my website: www.nutrition4health.com.au

PROTEINS

Food proteins are essential for healthy growth and repair. Once they are digested they become amino acids. Amino acids are raw materials for body proteins. We can think of amino acids as puzzle pieces, with the protein a completed puzzle. Essential amino acids, just like essential fatty acids, must be obtained from our diet. Adults need eight essential amino acids: valine, lysine, phenylalanine, tryptophan, isoleucine, leucine, methionine and threonine. The entire set of amino acids is easily obtained from meat muscle, including fish, poultry and eggs, and from dairy and soy products. Essential for healthy development, proteins also give our body the ability to repair itself, and to rebuild anything lost due to everyday wear and tear.

FIBRE

Fibre is indigestible plant matter. Fibre doesn't qualify for entry into the body, as it can't be absorbed by the digestive tract. It's what remains behind after the body has taken in all possible nutrients through the process of digestion. Far from being useless, however, this indigestible matter is what keeps the digestive tract fit. It helps to maintain a healthy gut flora. In addition, soluble fibre—found mostly in fruit, vegetables and certain grains—plays a role in filtering the digestive juices out of excess cholesterol. Good sources of fibre include wholemeal or wholegrain cereals, fruits and vegetables.

FLUID

The neglected nutrient, fluid is essential for our survival. Water is the optimal fluid, with unsweetened fruit juice, low-fat milk or soy beverage, tea and clear vegetable soups being other good choices. The need for fluid increases on hot days, and with physical exercise or fever. Aim to drink at least 2 litres (3.52 pints [UK], 4.23 pints [US]) of fluid a day, half of it as plain water.

Micronutrients

Micro means present in very small quantities. *Micronutrients* is the term used for vitamins and minerals. Vitamins and minerals are present in very small quantities in our foods, with some foods being much better sources than others. The way in which micronutrients work isn't fully understood, but it's clear that some are parts of body molecules which perform important functions in the body, and others are involved in regulating gene expression. One way of thinking about vitamins and minerals is as vital links in the chain of chemical communication in the overall manufacture of body goods.

You may like to spend some time going through Checkpoint 1 on the following pages to identify any weak spots in your diet.

The best food sources of vitamins and minerals

There is no substitute for organic—that is, naturally occurring—food nutrients. Inorganic forms of minerals and vitamins, like those present in numerous supplements, can be rather poorly absorbed.

Foods differ in the amounts and types of nutrients they contain, so it's useful to know which foods are the richest sources of the various nutrients. The 'Vitamin and mineral file' below provides a quick guide, along with some hints on how to avoid nutrients being lost during food preparation or dietary excesses.

checkpoint **1** *Spotting the missing nutrients in your diet*

To check if you could be low in the following vitamins, tick any of the foods or food groups listed in column two that are missing from or low in your diet.

Vitamin	Found in	How a vitamin deficiency may make you feel	Increases your need for intake of the vitamin
Vitamin B₁ (thiamin)	☐ Wholegrain cereals ☐ Nuts ☐ Peas, beans ☐ Beef, pork	• Irritable • Poor appetite • May lose weight	• Drinking alcohol • Heavy coffee consumption
Vitamin B₂ (riboflavin)	☐ Dairy products	• Sore mouth • Cracks in corners of mouth	• Drinking alcohol • Heavy exercise
Vitamin B₃ (niacin)	☐ Corn	• Irritable • Poor appetite • May lose weight	• Drinking alcohol
Vitamin B₆ (pyridoxine)	☐ Fish ☐ Lean meats, poultry ☐ Eggs ☐ Vegetables	• Deficiency is usually very rare	• Contraceptive pill
Vitamin B₁₂	☐ Eggs ☐ Milk ☐ Lean meats	• No early warning signs • Check blood chemistry	
Vitamin C	☐ Citrus fruit ☐ Fresh green vegetables	• Lethargic	• Cigarette smoking • Fever
Vitamin A	☐ Liver ☐ Dairy products ☐ Cold water fish	• Night blindness • Deficiency is usually rare	• Cigarette smoking
Vitamin D	☐ Butter, margarine ☐ Dairy ☐ Cold water fish ☐ Eggs	• Deficiency is usually rare	
Vitamin E	☐ Nuts, seeds ☐ Oils (soy, corn, cottonseed, wheat-germ, safflower)	• Not clear	• Polluted environment

Now for the minerals:

Mineral	Found in	How a mineral deficiency may make you feel	Increases your need for intake of the mineral
Iron	☐ Lean red meat ☐ Legumes ☐ Green vegetables	• Restless • Very fatigued • Weak • Poor concentration	• Pregnancy
Calcium	☐ Dairy products ☐ Fortified soy milk	• Trouble sleeping • Heart palpitations with prolonged deficiency	• Pregnancy • High caffeine intake • High salt intake
Zinc	☐ Seafood ☐ Lean meats ☐ Poultry	• Poor appetite • Changed sense of taste and smell	• Lactation • Some blood pressure pills
Copper	☐ Shellfish ☐ Nuts, seeds ☐ Legumes ☐ Fruit		• Heavy exercise
Selenium	☐ Fish, shellfish ☐ Lean red meat ☐ Onions, garlic ☐ Mushrooms ☐ Broccoli	• More frequent colds and flu	
Chromium	☐ May be low in a diet high in processed foods	• No clear physical symptoms	• Stress • Strenuous exercise • High sugar intake

How did you go? The fewer ticks you marked, the better. List below any vitamins or minerals your diet is low in, and then read the next section containing the 'Vitamin and mineral file'.

Vitamins: _____

Minerals: _____

Vitamin and mineral file

Vitamin A

Found in dairy products, eggs, sardines, herring, mackerel, margarine.

Pro vitamin A is found in dark green vegetables, deep yellow or orange vegetables, apricots, rockmelon (cantaloupe).

DON'T:

✗ Leave food exposed to air or sunlight.

✗ Cook food at temperatures above 100°C (212°F), for example, by frying.

Vitamin B$_1$

Found in wholegrain and enriched breads, marmite, vegemite, pork, lean meats and poultry, fish, legumes, nuts, green vegetables.

DON'T:

✗ Cook food in too much water.

✗ Soak food.

✗ Thaw food repeatedly or for a long time.

Vitamin B$_2$ (riboflavin)

Found in milk and dairy products, eggs, green leafy vegetables.

DON'T:

✗ Leave milk sitting out in the sun.

✗ Soak vegetables.

✗ Overcook food.

Vitamin B$_3$ (niacin)

Found in wholegrain and enriched cereals, legumes and nuts, lean meats, poultry, fish.

DON'T:

✖ Soak vegetables.

✖ Overcook food.

Vitamin B$_6$

Found in fish, lean poultry, lean meats, potatoes and sweet potatoes, vegetables.

DON'T:

✖ Cook food in too much water.

✖ Soak food.

✖ Thaw food repeatedly or for a long time.

Vitamin B$_{12}$

Found in low-fat milk and dairy products, fish, lean meats, lean poultry, eggs. Vitamin B$_{12}$ is made by microbes and isn't found in plant foods.

DON'T:

✖ Overcook your food.

Vitamin E

Found in wheatgerm, leafy vegetables (especially spinach), seeds and nuts (and oils from these), eggs, legumes.

DON'T:

✖ Leave food out in the open for a long time.

✖ Leave seeds, nuts or oils exposed to sunlight.

Vitamin C

Found in citrus fruits, tomatoes, strawberries, fresh green leafy vegetables, fresh peppers.

DON'T:

- Overcook food.
- Store food for long—eat it as fresh as possible.

Folate

Found in green leafy vegetables, oranges, orange juice, yeast extracts, peanuts, wholegrain cereals.

DON'T:

- Cook food in too much water.
- Soak food.
- Thaw food repeatedly or for a long time.
- Overcook food.

Calcium

Found in low-fat milk and dairy products, fortified soy beverages, salmon, sardines, broccoli, spinach.

DON'T:

- Eat too much protein.
- Eat too much salt.
- Drink too much coffee.

Copper

Found in shellfish, lean meats, legumes, nuts, wholegrain cereals.

Iron

Found in lean meats, lean poultry, tuna, salmon, wholegrains and cereals, legumes, dark green vegetables, prunes, dried apricots, raisins.

DON'T:

 Drink milk or eat dairy products with a meal rich in iron, as less iron will be absorbed.

Manganese

Found in legumes, nuts, wholegrain cereals.

Selenium

Found in lean meats and seafood, grains, cereals.

Zinc

Found in fish and seafood, lean meats, wheatgerm, nuts.

DON'T:

 Sprinkle raw bran over your food.

Bioavailability

Bioavailability refers to the ease of absorption of nutrients from the foods we ingest. Not all of the nutrients present in the digestive system are absorbed. Digestion is a dynamic process and the presence of other dietary constituents, or indeed other nutrients, either slows down or helps with the absorption of certain nutrients. The research on these interactions is still incomplete, but there are some very useful guidelines regarding the minerals iron, calcium and zinc.

COMPETING NUTRIENTS

While it's not true that we shouldn't mix one food group with another (an idea advocated by some diets), some food combinations are more beneficial than others. Put simply, it's a good idea to avoid mixing foods rich in competing nutrients. Competing nutrients are those that are absorbed into our bloodstream from the digestive system in the same way. If two or more competing nutrients are present in a meal, less of each of the nutrients will be absorbed due to the presence of the other. While sometimes this is unavoidable, we can make some easy adjustments to increase the absorption of three essential minerals, iron, calcium and zinc. Recent research has identified a number of dietary components that improve or inhibit absorption of these nutrients into our body. Let's consider the following case study.

Case study 1

It helps to stay informed

Alan is keen to take nutrition seriously as he would like to improve his well-being. He decided that he needs to lose some weight and get fitter, and as a result started to watch his fat intake and reduced his meal portions. Today, for lunch, he has ordered lean beef and vegetable stir-fry on steamed rice. To drink, he has chosen low-fat milk. Katie, Alan's girlfriend, is happy to go along with Alan's choice of meal, but she has chosen orange juice instead of milk.

Thinking about his meal as a source of iron and calcium, here's what Alan had:

• Beef—a rich source of iron.
• Low-fat milk—a rich source of calcium.

Calcium and iron compete with each other for absorption, as they enter the bloodstream from the digestive system in the same way. Hence, consuming both beef and milk together means that less of each mineral will be absorbed.

Now here's what Katie had:

- Beef—a rich source of iron.
- Orange juice—a rich source of vitamin C.

There is no rich source of calcium in Katie's meal. Therefore, she'll absorb more of the iron from her meal. In addition, she's having a beverage that's rich in vitamin C. Vitamin C increases the absorption of iron, so Katie will actually absorb more iron than if she ate the meal on its own without a drink.

You won't get stomach cramps from eating beef and drinking milk at the same time, as a healthy digestive system is designed to handle any food combinations. However, the following information isn't aimed at improving your *digestion*—it's aimed at improving your body's *nutritional status*. This is important in the following conditions:

- If you are anemic due to iron deficiency.
- If you are a vegetarian, and especially if you are a vegan and don't eat meat, poultry, fish, eggs or dairy products.
- If you are following a low-kilojoule diet to lose weight.

In all three cases above, and particularly if you eat a vegetarian diet, it's important to combine foods so as to optimise the absorption of iron, calcium and zinc. It's no coincidence that these three minerals are at risk in vegetarian diets, as their bioavailability is low in vegetables and other plant foods. The following section provides some guidelines on how to mix your foods and beverages to optimise the uptake of each of these nutrients.

GETTING MORE IRON, CALCIUM AND ZINC FROM YOUR DIET

Some important guidelines to note are:

- Eating foods containing iron is particularly important for girls, women, vegetarians and athletes.
- Eating foods containing calcium is particularly important for girls and women.
- Zinc is a nutrient that is relatively difficult to obtain from our diets, so increasing its absorption will help to provide our body with adequate amounts.

Guidelines for increasing absorption of iron, calcium and zinc

⇧ This symbol means absorption of the nutrient is increased when combined.

⇩ This symbol means absorption of the nutrient is decreased when combined.

Iron

⇧ vitamin C
⇧ muscle protein
⇩ phytic acid (present in raw bran, undercooked legumes)
⇩ polyphenols (found in tea, wine, herb teas, cocoa)
⇩ calcium

MEAL GUIDELINES TO INCREASE ABSORPTION OF IRON

✔ Drink unsweetened fruit juice or water with the meal.

✔ Avoid drinking cola, cocoa or milk.

✔ Include vegetables or fruit rich in vitamin C with the meal.

✔ Include some fish, chicken or meat with the meal.

Calcium

⬆ lactose (milk sugar)

⬇ phytic acid (present in raw bran, undercooked legumes)

⬇ saturated fats

⬇ iron

MEAL GUIDELINES TO INCREASE ABSORPTION AND RETENTION
OF CALCIUM

✔ Consume low-fat dairy products.

✔ Avoid drinking lots of coffee.

✔ Avoid using the salt shaker at the table.

✔ Cook with less salt.

✔ Consume alcohol in moderation.

✔ Avoid eating large quantities of meat.

Zinc

⬆ muscle protein

⬇ phytic acid (present in raw bran, undercooked legumes)

⬇ iron supplements

MEAL GUIDELINES TO INCREASE ABSORPTION OF ZINC

✓ Cook legumes well.

✓ Avoid eating raw bran. Instead use bran in baked goods such as bread or muffins.

✓ Include some fish, chicken or meat with the meal.

✓ If you need a zinc supplement, take it between meals with water to maximise absorption.

chapter two

Nutritional variety

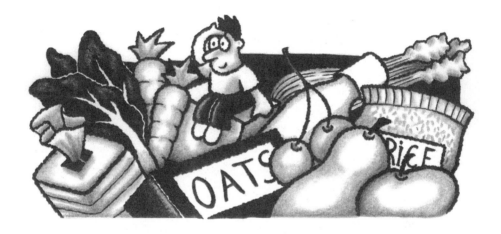

■ **GOALS**

- To include as many different foods in your day as possible
- To avoid eating the same food twice or more in the one day
- To change food choices from day to day

■ **BENEFITS**

- Variety prevents nutrient deficiencies
- It reduces the risk of food poisoning
- It prevents the development of food sensitivities

Variety in our food selection is the key principle of sound nutrition. Choosing a wide variety of foods helps to ensure that we consume all the nutrients necessary for good health. In addition, it reduces the risk of food poisoning and the development of food sensitivities.

Our grandparents and great-grandparents instinctively included a variety of foodstuffs in their daily diet. They were guided in their selection by what looked good, smelled good and felt good to the touch at their local greengrocer, butcher shop and fishmonger's. But in these days of supermarkets and highly processed and packaged foods, it's not so easy to be guided by the colour, smell and texture of foods. Instead, our choices are influenced by advertising and by packaging that may bear little relation to the food itself. As a result, we may eat a smaller variety of foods than is good for us.

Let's now look at some ways to assess the variety and quality of our daily food intake.

Working out your food variety score

Being far removed from selecting our food instinctively, one way of trying to meet our nutritional needs is to rely on scientific guidelines. Simply speaking, we should aim to eat at least twelve different foods every day. The more different foods we consume, the better our chances of nourishing our body with the entire team of nutrients essential for preserving health.

Here's how to work out your individual food variety score for a day. Count up all the individual foods that you ate and drank during one day. Count each food only once. For example, if you had pumpkin soup for lunch and baked pumpkin with your dinner, only count pumpkin once. If you had a salad for lunch, count each of the items that made up the salad (lettuce, snow peas, avocado, mushrooms and tomato, say), but only if each amounts to more than 2 tablespoons. Below is a sample daily food analysis to show you how it's done.

A sample daily food diary for assessing food variety

Wednesday		Score
Breakfast	toast, wholemeal X 2	1
	peanut butter, 2 tablespoons	1
	orange juice, 1 glass	1
Morning tea	vanilla yoghurt with acidophilus, 1 tub	1
Lunch	bread, white X 2	a
	ham, 1 slice	1
	tomato, slice	b
	flavoured fat-reduced milk, small carton	1
Afternoon tea	muesli bar	1
	apple	1
Dinner	steak, 120 g (4 oz)	1
	potato, 2 medium	1
	pumpkin, 1/2 cup	1
	broccoli, 1/2 cup	1
	gravy, 3 tablespoons	1
Total score		12

a Repeated item therefore no score—both white and wholemeal breads are made from wheat.
b Quantities smaller than 2 tablespoons (except for fats, oils and yeast extracts) don't represent a sufficient quantity to rate as a score, for example, a slice of tomato in a sandwich, two olives or less than 2 tablespoons of salad dressing in a salad.

Now do the same and total your score. How did you go? A score of over 12 daily is considered excellent. You may like to continue keeping a food diary for seven days to work out your weekly variety score. Aim for a weekly score of between 20 and 30 to meet your essential nutrient requirements. Use the following table to help you work out your daily or weekly variety score.

BIOLOGICALLY DISTINCT FOOD GROUPS

1. Eggs (all varieties)

Dairy

2. Milk, ice-cream, cheese

Live cultures

3. Yoghurt (e.g. acidophilus, bifidobacteria)

Yeast

4. Vegemite, marmite

Fish (incl. canned)

5. Fatty fish (tuna, anchovies, salmon, sardines, herring, mackerel, kippers)
6. Salt water fish
7. Fresh water fish
8. Fish roe (caviar salad)
9. Shellfish (mussels, oysters, squid)
10. Crustaceans (prawns, lobster)

Meat

11. Ruminants (lamb, beef, veal)
12. Monogastric (pork, ham, bacon)
13. Poultry (chicken, duck, turkey)
14. Game (quail, wild duck, pigeon)
15. Game (kangaroo, rabbit)
16. Liver

17. Brain
18. All other organ meats

Legumes (incl. canned)

19. Peas (fresh, dried, split peas); chickpeas (dried, roasted); beans (haricot, kidney, lima, broad); lentils (red, brown, green); soy products (tofu, milk).

Cereals

20. Wheat (bread, pasta, ready-to-eat)
21. Corn (cornflakes, polenta)
22. Barley (bread, barley cereal)
23. Oats (porridge, cereal, bread)
24. Rye (bread, ready-to-eat)
26. Rice (grain, ready-to-eat)
27. Other grains (millet, linseed)

Fats and oils

28. Oils
29. Hard/soft spreads

Beverages

30. Water (incl. mineral)
31. Tea, coffee, herbal teas, wine, beer, spirits

Fermented foods

32. Miso, tempeh, soy sauce

33. Sauerkraut

34. All other varieties

Sugar/confectionary

35. All varieties (incl. soft drinks)

Vegetables (incl. canned and frozen)

36. Root (potato, carrot, sweet potato, beetroot, parsnip, bamboo shoot, ginger, radish, water chestnut)

37. Flowers (broccoli, cauliflower)

38. Stalks (celery, asparagus)

39. Onion (spring, garlic, leeks)

40. Tomatoes, okra

41. Beans (green, snow peas)

42. Leafy greens (spinach, silverbeet, endive, kale, chicory, parsley, lettuce)

43. Peppers (capsicum, chillies)

44. Marrow (zucchini, squash, cucumber, turnip, eggplant, swede, pumpkin)

45. Fungi (e.g. mushrooms)

46. Herbs/spices

Nuts and seeds

47. Almond, cashew, chestnut, coconut, hazelnut, peanuts, peanut butter, pine nut, pistachio, pumpkin seed, sesame seed, tahini, walnut

Fruit

48. Stone (peach, cherry, plums, apricot, avocado, olive, prune)

49. Apples

50. Pears, nashi

51. Berries (strawberries)

52. Grapes (incl. raisins, sultanas)

53. Bananas

54. Citrus (orange, lemon)

55. Melon (honeydew, watermelon)

56. Kiwi, date, passionfruit

57. Tropical (mango, pineapple)

Source: G.S. Savige, B. Hsu-hage, and M.L. Wahlqvist, 'Food variety as nutritional therapy', *Current Therapeutics*, March 1997, pp. 57–67; http://health.med.monash.edu.au/healthyeating/variety

Using colour as a measure of food variety

One way to increase the variety of food you eat is to include different-coloured foods at every meal. If your meal is predominantly of one colour (say, shades of brown), not only will it look rather drab but it won't provide you with a wide variety of nutrients either. Ideally, what's on your plate or in your bowl should include a mixture of different colours—the more the better, as each colour represents a certain mixture of nutrients with specific nutrients dominating. You could say that nutrients are colour-coded.

The box below provides an example of how this works.

Are they different or the same?

Picture in your mind a hot meat pie with a dollop of tomato sauce on top. Now picture a bowl of steaming spaghetti bolognaise. Because it looks and smells different from the meat pie, you might think they are different foods. You might think that if you had a pie for lunch and spaghetti bolognaise for dinner, you would be varying your food intake. However, if we look at the main ingredients in these foods, we find they are both made with beef, onions, tomatoes, flour and fat. Thus, they have an almost identical nutrient profile, and differ only in the actual amounts (not types) of nutrients.

If you think of these two foods in terms of colour, you can easily see that although they might be different 'foods', they are the same colours (brown, red and cream) and thus have a very similar nutrient profile.

Incidentally, spaghetti bolognaise is a lower fat option and therefore a healthier choice. We will look at fats in more detail later.

If you eat two meals on the same day with similar ingredients, you'll reduce your chances of getting all the essential nutrients. No one food or food group can provide all the nutrients essential for good health. Variety is the key.

Using models to illustrate optimum nutritional variety

There are a number of models that illustrate the concept of nutritional variety and one of these is the healthy eating pyramid. The concept of the model is simple. Foods are divided into individual food groups and are arranged in the form of a pyramid.

HEALTHY EATING PYRAMID

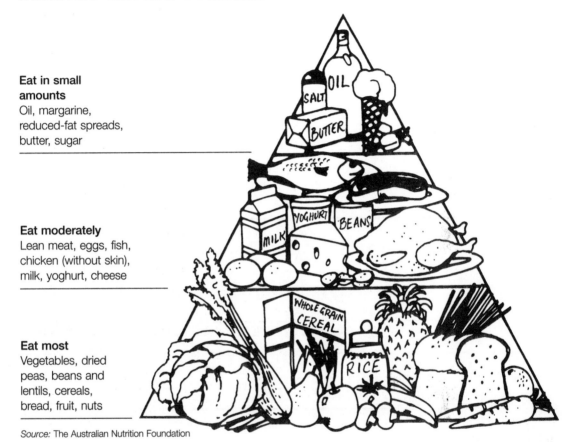

Eat in small amounts
Oil, margarine, reduced-fat spreads, butter, sugar

Eat moderately
Lean meat, eggs, fish, chicken (without skin), milk, yoghurt, cheese

Eat most
Vegetables, dried peas, beans and lentils, cereals, bread, fruit, nuts

Source: The Australian Nutrition Foundation

Foods forming the base of the pyramid are to be eaten more often, and in larger serves, than the foods at the top.

The 12345+ Food and Nutrition Plan, developed by the Human Division Unit at CSIRO Australia, may be even more helpful, as it shows the minimum recommended number of serves for each food group within the pyramid model. (I believe that up to two serves daily of lean meat or a low-fat alternative is acceptable.) Take some time to look at this model. How does it apply to your daily diet?

THE 12345+ FOOD AND NUTRITION PLAN

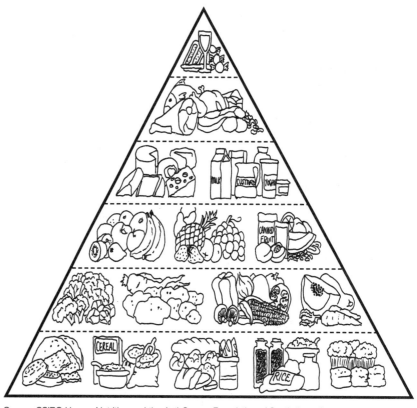

Source: CSIRO Human Nutrition and the Anti-Cancer Foundation of South Australia

Now take a look at Checkpoint 2.

checkpoint **2** *Assessing food variety in your diet using food groups*

Go back to the list you made of all the foods you ate and drank in one day. Place each of the foods and drinks into one of the five food groups listed below. Don't include tea, coffee and water, but do count milk and other drinks. (Refer to either of the models given above to work out how to allocate the items you consumed to the various food groups.)

Basic food groups

Fruit and vegetables	Total no. of serves:* ___
Grains and cereals	Total no. of serves: ___
Meat and alternatives	Total no. of serves: ___
Dairy products	Total no. of serves: ___
Fats (indulgences)	Total no. of serves: ___

Look at the table below to work out how much of each food is a serve.

Now write your scores in the spaces here.

Fruit and vegetables	___ / 7 (recommended number)
Grains and cereals	___ / 5 to 12
Meat and alternatives	___ / 1 to 2
Dairy products	___ / 2 to 3
Fats (indulgences)	___ / 1 to 2

Individual food serves in the five food groups

Fruit & vegetables	Grains & cereals	Lean meat & alternatives	Dairy & soy	Examples of Indulgences
• 1 medium piece of fruit	• 1 slice of bread	• 60–100 g (2–3½ oz) lean cooked meat	• 1 glass of milk	• 1 medium piece plain cake
• 3 small fruit (e.g. apricot)	• 1 small or half a large roll	• Half a cup lean mince	• 200 g (7 oz) tub of yoghurt	• 1 bun
• Half a medium melon	• 1 English muffin	• 2 small lamb chops	• 40 g (1⅖ oz) slice of cheese	• 1 small piece rich cake
• 20 grapes or cherries	• 1 scone	• 2 slices roast meat	• 1 glass of fortified soy milk	• 1 small piece pastry
• 1 cup of berry fruits	• 1 cup cooked pasta	• 2 eggs		• 2–3 sweet biscuits
• 2 tablespoons sultanas	• Half a cup cooked rice	• 100 g (3½ oz) cooked fish		• 2 scoops ice-cream
• 1 medium potato	• Half a cup cooked couscous	• 100 g (3½ oz) poultry		• Half a chocolate bar
• Half a cup green vegetables	• 30–40 g (1–1⅗ oz) breakfast cereal	• Two-thirds cup cooked legumes		• 30 g (1 oz) toffees
• One-third cup carrots, pumpkin, peas, corn, eggplant, squash	• One-third cup muesli			• 30 g (1 oz) crisps (1 small packet)
	• Half a cup cooked porridge			• One-third meat pie
				• Half a sausage roll

Source: CSIRO and the Anti-Cancer Foundation of South Australia, 1992

How did you go? Aim to adjust the number of serves for each food group in your diet to meet the recommended number. Use the table on the previous page to keep track of your serves for each food group.

chapter three

Nutritional supplements

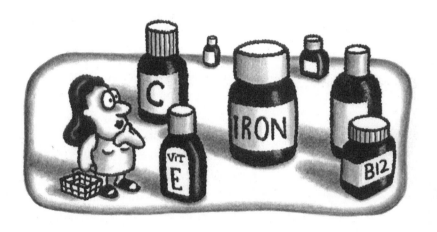

■ GOAL

- To recognise which, if any, supplements to take, when and in what amounts

■ BENEFITS

- When diet is inadequate, supplements prevent nutrient deficiencies

- You will prevent side effects caused by taking supplements in toxic amounts

- You will save money by not buying useless supplements

The variety of nutritional supplements is immense, and to list and consider them all is beyond the scope of this book. There are, however, some useful guidelines to consider when buying supplements and, indeed, some safety measures we need to take. The production and promotion of nutritional supplements is big business, and it is useful to keep in mind that, at the end of the day, it is not always your health that is foremost in the minds of the manufacturers. Big claims and promises are made for many supplements: some are promoted as having the ability to heal just about any ailment under the sun. In reality, only a fraction of nutritional supplements have scientific backing for their use—that is, after being tested in an objective way on a significant number of people, shown to have health benefits. For most nutrients, supplementation is useful only if your diet is lacking in that particular nutrient.

Before you start taking any nutritional supplement, remember that they fall outside the regulatory area of bodies such as the Australia and New Zealand Food Authority and the Therapeutic Goods Administration. Therefore, companies that produce nutritional supplements are not required by those bodies to limit the health claims made for the supplements or to prove that their claims are legitimate. *Don't believe everything you read. Be wary of supplements that claim to cure every ailment under the sun. They are a waste of money.* There are, however, times when supplements can be helpful.

Preventing or correcting nutrient deficiencies

Supplementation can be helpful at times when your diet is lacking balance, or when your body's needs have increased and it is more difficult to obtain all nutrients from your diet alone. The following situations are examples of times when you may need supplements:

- You suffer from frequent colds.
- You are recovering from the flu.
- You are losing weight on a diet of less than 6000 kilojoules (1400 calories) a day.
- You have a poor appetite.
- During periods of stress.
- You are travelling overseas, where your diet may be compromised.

Various lifestyle habits also create a greater need for some nutrients. For example:

- Drinking alcohol in excess of three drinks a week increases the body's need for vitamins B_1, B_6, A and D, folate and beta-carotene.
- Smoking increases the body's need for vitamins B_6, C and E, folate and beta-carotene.
- The oral contraceptive pill increases the body's need for vitamins B_6, folate and beta-carotene.
- Vegetarianism—when the diet excludes meat, poultry and fish it may be low in vitamins B_{12} and D.

If any of the above lifestyle habits apply to you, it may be useful to take a supplementary form of the appropriate nutrients. Except in cases of a few chronic conditions that we will look at shortly, it is best to take nutritional supplements in dosages approximating the recommended dietary intake (see the following table).

The usual method for determining if nutrient stores and levels are low is by a blood test. If you suspect that you are suffering from a nutrient deficiency, you can ask your doctor to

Approximately 40 countries have recommendations in place for the optimum daily consumption of nutrients. Official recommendations for this daily intake vary from country to country as each country has its own nutrient standards set out by the relevant expert communities. In Australia, the recommended nutrient intakes are set by the National Health and Medical Research Council (NH&MRC) and are termed 'Recommended Dietary Intakes' or RDIs. In the United States the term 'Recommended Daily Allowances' (RDAs) is the equivalent and Recommended Daily Amounts are used in the United Kingdom.

Recommended dietary intakes (RDIs) for adults from Australia,* the USA and the UK, respectively

Nutrient	Men (19–64 years)	Women (19–54 years)
Vitamin A	750/1000/750 mcg retinol equivalents	750/800/750 mcg retinol equivalents
Vitamin B$_1$ (thiamin)	1.1/1.5/0.9–1.3 mg	0.8/1.1/0.7–0.9 mg
Vitamin B$_2$ (riboflavin)	1.7/1.7/1.7 mg	1.2/1.3/1.3 mg
Vitamin B$_3$ (niacin)	18–20/19/6.6[†] mg niacin equivalents	12–14/15/6.6[†] mg niacin equivalents
Vitamin B$_6$ (pyridoxine)	1.3–1.9 mg/2.0 mg/15 ug[§]	0.9–1.4 mg/1.6 mg/15 ug[§]
Total folate	200/200/300 mcg	200/180/300 mcg
Vitamin B$_{12}$	2.0/2.0/– mcg	2.0/2.0/– mcg
Vitamin C	40/60/30 mg	30/60/30 mg
Vitamin E	10/10/– mg alpha tocopherol equivalents	7/8/– mg alpha tocopherol equivalents
Calcium	800/1000/500 mg	800/1000/500 mg
Iron	7/10/10 mg	12–16/10–15/12 mg
Magnesium	320/420/– mg	270/320 – mg
Phosphorus	1000/700/– mg	1000/700/– mg
Potassium	1950–5460/–/– mg	1950–5460/–/– mg
Selenium	85/70/– mcg	70/55/– mcg
Zinc	12/12/– mg	12/12/– mg

Notes: [†] per 1000 Kcal (4200 kg) for all age groups

[§] per g of protein for anyone above 1 year of age

* Source: A.S. Truswell (ed.) *The Recommended Nutrient Intakes: Australian Papers*, Sydney: Australian Professional Publications, 1990

arrange a blood test and to prescribe supplements for you. In addition, refer back to Checkpoint 1, in the section on micronutrients in Chapter 1, if you are deficient in any nutrient—in particular, iron and zinc. Iron and zinc are poorly absorbed from supplements, and you will need to plan your diet carefully to increase your consumption of these minerals.

Reducing the risk of chronic conditions

Recent scientific investigations into the benefits derived from supplements in excess of the RDI have shown some positive results in the prevention of a few chronic conditions. These chronic conditions are:

- *Osteoporosis:* High dosages of calcium have been found to be beneficial in stopping bone thinning.
- *Heart disease:* High dosages of vitamin E have been associated with a lower incidence of heart disease, most likely through the vitamin's action as an antioxidant. (Antioxidants are discussed in Chapter 6.) However, researchers note that antioxidants work synergistically and a balanced diet is advantageous over a single antioxidant supplement.
- *Arthritis:* Supplementation with essential fatty acids—namely w-3 fatty acids EPA and DHA—have been found to be beneficial in reducing both inflammation and the pain associated with inflammatory changes.

As the dosages needed to elicit these beneficial effects are far in excess of the RDI, the taking of supplements in these therapeutic doses is best supervised by a general practitioner.

Safety concerns and safety margins

Some nutritional supplements if taken in excess will cause side effects. The following guide will help you to determine whether you are taking any supplement in excess of its safe upper intake limit.

VITAMIN AND MINERAL SUPPLEMENTS

Some minerals and vitamins can be toxic if taken in large amounts. Taking supplements in quantities which exceed safe upper limits for these nutrients has been shown to produce a variety of symptoms, and in some cases has resulted in severe sickness. Numerous studies have identified a wide range of symptoms. If you are taking any supplements, have a look at Checkpoint 3 to determine whether you are taking them in harmful doses. If you find that you *are* taking any supplements in doses exceeding their safety limit, discontinue or reduce the dosage of the supplement unless, in the rare case, it was prescribed by your doctor. Check all supplements to see if you are taking a combined dosage that is above the safe upper limit. *Your supplement should ideally offer the nutrient in a dose close to its RDI.*

checkpoint **3**

Checking whether you are taking a harmful dose of supplements

Some vitamins and minerals can be toxic if taken in excess. Are you taking more than is safe? If you take any of the vitamin or mineral supplements listed in the following tables, write down the amounts you are taking in the relevant columns, then check them against their safe upper levels. The figures given are for adults only and should not be used as guidelines for pregnant women and children.

Safe upper levels for vitamins and minerals that can be toxic

Vitamin/Mineral	My dose	Safe upper level (daily)
A	_____	3000 mcg
D	_____	50 mcg
E	_____	400 mg
Nicotinic acid[a]	_____	< 500 mg
Pyridoxine	_____	100 mg
B_{12}	_____	No upper limit
C	_____	2 g
B-carotene	_____	No upper limit[b]
Folate	_____	1000 mcg
Chromium picolinate	_____	< 1000 mcg
Chromium hexavalent	_____	< 335 mcg for 70 kg person
Selenium	_____	200 mcg
Iodine	_____	1000 mcg
Zinc	_____	15 mg

Notes: [a] Unless supervised by a doctor.
[b] Yellow skin pigmentation is a side effect of intakes >30 mg B-carotene daily. This is not harmful.

MISCELLANEOUS SUPPLEMENTS

There is a wide variety of supplements or pseudo-supplements available beyond the nutritional supplements. Protein powders, herbal mixtures, oils, and numerous other concoctions fill the shelves in health food stores, chemists and supermarkets. In most cases, there is no reliable scientific evidence for their claimed benefits. Although for most people these supplements are safe, some people may experience side effects ranging from mild discomfort to rare, but life-threatening, allergic reactions. Discuss your supplements with your doctor or nutritionist, so that you are aware of both the benefits and the risks.

part two

Prevention is better than cure

chapter four

Keeping fit

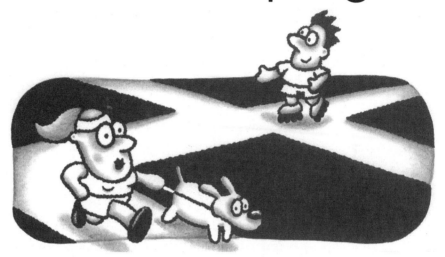

■ GOALS

- To lower your weight to an ideal weight for your height, if the weight loss needed is less than 6 kilograms (14 pounds)

- To lower your weight by 10 per cent of your body weight otherwise

- To maintain or reduce your waist to hip ratio to below 0.8 if you are a woman

- To maintain or reduce your waist to hip ratio to below 0.95 if you are a man

■ BENEFITS

- You will have improved fitness and athletic power

- Your energy levels will increase

- You will have higher self-esteem

- Your looks will be improved

- You will enjoy your physical health for longer and ward off heart disease, diabetes and high blood pressure

Too much weight can get in your way. It will slow you down and you will feel tired faster. It may also make you feel frustrated and low about yourself. Most important of all, it will burden your health. By keeping your weight in the healthy weight range and keeping fit, you will help to avoid these problems.

Food—our source of energy

With the exception of water, every food we consume has stored energy. The amount of stored energy depends on the composition of the food—that is, the amounts of fat, carbohydrate, protein or alcohol it contains. All four of these components are sources of energy that can be harnessed by our body once they have been digested. We can measure how much energy a food provides by combusting the food in a perfectly sealed vessel suspended in water, and then measuring the increase in temperature of the water. The higher the energy content of the food, the higher the temperature rise. The energy of a particular food is measured in kilojoules. The energy content, given in kilojoules per gram, for pure fat, carbohydrate, protein and alcohol is as follows:

Fat	37 kilojoules, or 9 calories
Carbohydrate	16 kilojoules, or 4 calories
Protein	17 kilojoules, or 4 calories
Alcohol	29 kilojoules, or 7 calories

As you can see, fats provide over twice the amount of energy provided by carbohydrates and proteins, with alcohol not far behind. While the main function of fats and carbohydrates is to provide energy, the main function of protein is to repair the body. Only if protein is consumed in excess of what is needed for growth and reconstruction work—for example, the repair of injured tissues—will it be used as fuel in the form of sugar. Adults need relatively less protein than children, who are growing rapidly, yet typically the daily diet of an adult in Western society is high in protein, and excess protein contributes extra kilojoules.

Although it is useful to estimate the energy content of foods, we need to look at the bigger picture. We need to consider how much of the stored energy in the foods we eat is actually available for use. Numerous studies looking at the process of digestion have led to the following conclusion: not all kilojoules are the same. To be more scientifically correct, *our body needs to do more work to get energy from carbohydrates and proteins than it does from fats and alcohol.* The digestion of carbohydrates and proteins requires a bigger initial energy investment (or loss). This investment is the energy required to digest and assimilate the food before the food energy can be used. In practice, then, carbohydrate- and protein-rich foods supply us with fewer kilojoules than we find listed in the food tables. This is one of the reasons why I don't recommend kilojoule counting for the purposes of losing weight.

Energy content of carbohydrate-rich food – energy used for digestion
= energy available for use

The energy required for the digestion, absorption and assimilation of any food is called dietary-induced thermogenesis. This is the amount of energy our body loses in order to use the food energy later. The energy used up for dietary-induced thermogenesis varies between individuals; just like fuel efficiency varies between car models. Estimates available from past research indicate losses of between 10 and 35 per cent of the stored food energy.

At present it is impossible to measure the energy loss due to dietary-induced thermogenesis for any one person. What *is* known is that every time we eat, our body burns a little extra energy to assimilate the food, and *we burn more of it if our diet is rich in carbohydrates and/or proteins rather than fats or alcohol.*

Energy balance

The energy derived from the food we consume allows us to go about our daily activities. It is utilised in limitless chemical reactions to maintain our health and keep our cells in top shape. Without adequate food energy we would eventually cease to go about these activities, just like a battery-operated toy stops working once the batteries run out. Our energy intake isn't constant, however, and, unlike a battery-operated toy which needs a certain amount of voltage to work at all, we can continue to function even if we eat less than our energy needs for some time. This is because the body is able to store food energy for just such times of low energy intake.

The principal energy storage sites in the body are the muscles, liver and adipose tissue (fat stores). The muscles and liver store energy as glycogen. Glycogen in the liver is the sugar jar in our body. It's the source of quickly available energy in the form of sugar or glucose. Glycogen is a small fuel reserve and runs out within days. Adipose tissue, on the other hand, is a much bigger and longer-lasting source of energy, sufficient to last for at least a month.

On any particular day, our body can be in a positive or a negative energy balance. If the food you have eaten today has provided you with more energy than your body has used to keep you going, including carrying out all your daily activities, you are in a *positive energy balance*—that is, you have increased your energy stores or, in simple terms, you have put on weight. If the reverse is true and you have eaten less energy than you used up, this puts you in a *negative energy balance*. The extra energy you needed came from your energy stores; therefore, you have lost weight.

The day-to-day changes in weight are very small and hardly noticeable. Chronic undereating, however, will result in significant weight loss, just as chronic overeating will result in significant weight gain.

> In Western countries, overeating—eating in excess of our energy needs—results in obesity, a significant health problem.

Preserve your health— avoid overeating

The latest scientific data on the process of aging suggest that a healthy, active lifestyle can lengthen your life by ten years simply by keeping your body weight in a healthy weight range. Scientific research shows that overeating increases the production of free radicals. Free radicals are extremely reactive molecules that damage cell structures, causing premature aging. Reducing your kilojoule intake if you are overweight will therefore not only lead to weight loss, but will also preserve your well-being for longer.

People's energy needs differ

Energy needs differ from one person to the next. We all know of people who can eat like a horse without ever seeming to gain

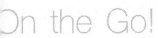

weight, and of others who say they only have to *smell* food and they start piling on the kilograms. It's a pointless, even soul-destroying, exercise to compare our own energy needs with other people's.

We all need different amounts of energy, because the rate at which we burn energy is different. The rate at which we burn energy is called our metabolic rate. Our metabolic rate is influenced by our:

- *Gender:* Men have a higher metabolic rate than women, as they have a relatively higher muscle mass.
- *Muscle mass:* A woman with good muscle tone has a higher metabolic rate than a woman with relatively small muscle mass.
- *Activity level:* Active people keep their metabolic rate up through regular exercise and on average have a higher rate than do sedentary individuals.
- *Genes:* Genetic influences regulate the metabolic rate to some extent.
- *Food intake:* Crash diets lower the metabolic rate.
- *Age:* As we age, our metabolic rate slows down. The process is very gradual, but over a period of years it becomes noticeable. This is one reason why people gain weight as they get older.
- *Thyroid activity:* The thyroid gland is responsible for the hormones that control our metabolic rate. A 'slow thyroid' (a condition where the thyroid gland fails to produce sufficient amounts of thyroxine, a hormone which regulates the metabolic rate) reduces the metabolic rate.

Whatever your metabolic rate is, you can increase it by increasing the amount of exercise you do, by eating less at a time but more frequently, or by taking medication if your thyroid is slow. (Medication must only be taken under medical supervision.)

Estimating your energy needs

Your gender, age, activity level and genetic make-up are the main determinants of your current energy needs. From time to time, other factors will influence your daily energy needs—for example, fever and exposure to extreme temperatures can increase your energy needs significantly. However, these conditions are rare and working out your average energy needs is of more use. If you are in good health and the temperature conditions aren't extreme, you can calculate your average daily energy needs by following the steps set out in the box below.

Calculating your average daily energy needs

Remember: 1000 kilojoules = 1 megajoule (1 MJ) = 238 calories

Step 1: Find your basal metabolic rate (BMR) from the table below. Just put your weight in kilograms into the formula that matches your age bracket. You will get your daily energy needs in megajoules (MJ). Multiply this figure by 1000 to get your BMR in kilojoules.

Estimating basal metabolic rate:
your energy expenditure while on standby

Gender	Age bracket (years)	Formula[a]
		Weight must be in kilograms! 1 kilogram = 2.3 pounds
Male	18–30	0.063 × weight + 2.896
	30–60	0.048 × weight + 3.653
	Over 60	0.049 × weight + 2.459
Female	18–30	0.062 × weight + 2.036
	30–60	0.034 × weight + 3.538
	Over 60	0.038 × weight + 2.755

Note: [a] Formula taken from W.N. Schofield, C. Schofield and W.P.T. James 'Basal metabolic rate: review and prediction, together with an annotated bibliography of source material', *Human Nutrition Clinical Nutrition*, no. 39C (Suppl.1), 1985, pp.1–96.
Source: A.S. Truswell (ed.) *Recommended Nutrient Intakes: Australian Papers*, Sydney: Australian Professional Publications, 1990.

Your BMR is the energy you use while you are 'on standby'—that is, it's the energy you would use up if you were to sleep 24 hours a day, using energy solely for activities controlled by the autonomic system, such as breathing, maintaining your heartbeat, and so on.

Step 2: You now need to consider the energy you use for any physical activities. Work out your activity level from the table below.

Working out your activity level

Activity level	Multiply your BMR by	
Choose from	Men	Women
Sedentary		
No exercise	1.4	1.4
Light		
Table tennis, golf, ten-pin bowling	1.5	1.5
Moderate		
Cycling (slow pace), cricket, sailing, swimming (slow pace), tennis (moderate pace)	1.8	1.7
Heavy		
Tennis (fast pace), roller-skating, swimming (moderate pace), aerobics, basketball, football, jogging, squash, weight training	2.1	1.8
Very heavy		
Race swimming, race rowing, race cycling, fast squash, running (10–15 km/hour or 6⅕–9⅓ miles/hour)	2.3	2.0

Source: A.S. Truswell (ed.) *Recommended Nutrient Intakes: Australian Papers*, Sydney: Australian Professional Publications, 1990.

Step 3: Now multiply your BMR _____ (converted to kilojoules) by your activity level _____ to get _____ kilojoules.

Consider any relevant extras from the following:

- If you are pregnant and in your second or third trimester: add 1000 kilojoules.
- If you are breast-feeding: add 2400 kilojoules.

Overall, your daily energy needs are: _____ kilojoules.

You may like to visit the website www.nutrition4health.com.au to calculate your energy needs and to find individual recommendations for a healthy weight.

If you are gaining weight, it means that your energy intake exceeds your energy needs. Your body stores the surplus food energy as body energy stores (fat), to be used later. The end result is that you put on weight. The most common reason for putting on weight is eating too much fat. This may or may not be coupled with too much sugar and/or alcohol. *If you want to lose weight, start by targeting fat.*

Four golden rules for weight loss

✔ Avoid using a lot of oil or butter when preparing meals at home, and choose meals that are low in fat when eating out. You'll find many useful guidelines on low-fat dining, and eating out in general, in the appendix section of this book. Now is a good time to tackle the quiz in Checkpoint 4. Put your diet to the test, and then follow the guidelines on how to cut back on your intake of fat.

✔ Look at your meal pattern. Do you skip meals, only to find yourself snacking on greasy convenience foods or a chocolate bar? By delaying or skipping meals, you are also slowing down your metabolic rate.

✓ Get into the habit of eating regular meals at least three times a day. Regular low-fat snacks in between your main meals may take care of any pre-meal cravings. And remember that being on a low-fat diet doesn't mean feeling tired, as carbohydrates provide us with a steady supply of energy.

✓ *It's most important that the changes you make to your diet are long-lasting.* You will be far better off making smaller changes that you can live with, rather than radical sacrifices for just a week or two. The result will be long-term weight control.

checkpoint **4**

How much fat do you eat?

Circle your answers, add up the scores and then refer to the comments at the end of this checkpoint. Good luck!

Question	Score

1. Do you trim fat off meats and remove chicken skin prior to cooking?

Never	4
Sometimes	3
Mostly	2
Always	1

2. How is your main meal usually cooked?

Deep-fried	5
Pan-fried or shallow-fried	4
Roasted with added fat	3
Roasted with no added fat or dry pan-fried	2
Grilled	0
Boiled/steamed/microwaved	0

3. Do you add margarine/butter/white sauce/gravy/sour cream to your meals?

Always	2
Occasionally	1
Never	0

4. What desserts do you usually have?

Pastries or pies	2
Cheesecake or mousse	2
Fruit and cream	1
Fruit and ice-cream/custard	1
Fruit	0
Nothing	0

5. How many times a week do you eat takeaway 'fast' foods (e.g. pizza, fish and chips, burgers)?

Every day	4
3–5	3
1–2	2
Less than once a week	1
Never	0

6. What cereals do you usually have for breakfast?

Toasted muesli	2
Plain muesli	1
Plain cereals with less than 5 g of fat per 100 g (⅙ oz per 3½ oz)	0
Porridge or instant oats	0

7. What type of milk or soy beverage do you usually use?

Full cream or regular	2
Fat-reduced milks	1
Low-fat milk (e.g. skim)	0

8. For a cooked breakfast, you would have:

Bacon/sausage and fried eggs	3
Trimmed bacon and lean sausage and dry-fried egg	2
Boiled/poached egg and grilled tomato	1
Grilled tomato/baked beans/creamed corn/spaghetti	0

9. How often do you eat sausages, salami, pate, processed cold meats (e.g. chicken roll)?

At least once a day	4
3–5 times a week	3
1–2 times a week	2
Less than once a week	1
Never	0

10. How often do you snack on any or all of the following:
    chips, crisps, cheddar cheese, nuts, Jatz?

At least once a day	4
3–5 times a week	3
1–2 times a week	2
Less than once a week	1
Never	0

11. How often do you snack on any or all of the following: chocolate,
    carob bars, chocolate- or cream-filled biscuits, pastries, cakes?

At least once a day	4
3–5 times a week	3
1–2 times a week	2
Less than once a week	1
Never	0

12. How do you spread your margarine or butter ?

Thickly	3
Medium—just covering the bread	2
Thin—just a scraping on the bread	1
None at all	0

13. What dressing do you usually add to salads?

Regular mayonnaise	2
Regular French or Italian dressing or home-made with oil	2
Low-fat mayonnaise (e.g. 97% fat-free)	0
No oil dressings	0
Lemon juice and herbs	0

14. How many times a week would you eat fatty cheese (e.g. cheddar
    or cream cheese)?

At least once a day	4
3–5 times a week	3
1–2 times a week	2
Less than once a week	1
Never	0

YOUR TOTAL SCORE   ——

How you scored

1–10   That's great! You are keeping the fat content of your diet nice and low.

11–16   That's not too bad. However, there is room for improvement. You could do with some 'spring cleaning'. For some great suggestions, see 'Suggestions for spring cleaning your diet' following.

17+   You've got some serious repair work to do on your present diet. Read carefully 'Suggestions for spring cleaning your diet' following.

Suggestions for spring cleaning your diet

Go back over your answers and circle below the questions where you picked up more than one point. Then note the changes you need to make in your diet.

Question 1

- Always trim fat from meat and remove the skin from chicken. To save time, consider buying fillets or trimmed cuts of meat, such as new-fashioned pork or lamb.

Question 2

- Keep deep-frying and shallow-frying to just twice a week at the most—less often if you are overweight.
- When roasting, place meat on a rack and place a tray below it to collect the dripping fat.
- Don't cook vegetables in fat. Instead, brush them with a small amount of oil using a pastry brush, wrap in foil and bake in the oven.
- Cook your meal by grilling, microwaving, poaching in stock and herbs, or boiling (as in soups and casseroles) without adding any fat.

Question 3

- Don't add any butter, margarine, fatty sauces, gravy or sour cream to your meals.

Question 4

• Low-fat tasty dessert ideas: fruit salad, fruit and low-fat ice-cream, fruit and low-fat yoghurt, warm fruit compotes in winter.

Question 5

• Limit takeaway food to less than once a week.
• Lower-fat takeaway meal suggestions: roasted chicken (remove skin and choose breast or leg), corn on the cob and bread roll (e.g. at Red Rooster); vegetarian pizza with less cheese—ask for a light coat of cheese only; grilled burgers without cheese or mayonnaise.

Question 6

• Avoid toasted muesli or any other toasted cereal.
• When buying cereal, choose ones with less than 5 per cent fat.

Question 7

• Choose fat-reduced milk or skim milk in place of regular cow's milk.
• Choose fat-reduced soy beverages.

Question 8

Some great low-fat hot breakfast suggestions:
• Grilled tomato and baked beans
• Grilled tomato and braised mushrooms
• Grilled tomato, creamed corn and asparagus
• Any combination of the above

Alternatively:
• Choose eggs that are boiled, poached or scrambled by dry-frying.
• Limit eggs to about four a week if your cholesterol level is high or you are overweight.

Question 9

• Use lean ham (e.g. soccerball, ham deluxe, shaved ham), shaved chicken, or 97 per cent fat-free cold cuts on your sandwiches.

Question 10

• Choose unbuttered popcorn, rice crackers with salsa, or cruskets with cottage or ricotta cheese for snacks.

Question 11

• Choose plain, fruit biscuits, low-fat fruit muffins, low-fat yoghurt or low-fat fruit smoothies for your snacks.

Question 12

• An easy way to cut back on fat is to give up spreading butter or margarine on your bread. You may like to use mustards, horseradish, low-fat hummus, low-fat mayonnaise or tzadziki instead.

Question 13

• Make a fantastic dressing of fresh herbs and some spices, and add lemon juice or balsamic vinegar (or both) for great flavour without fat.
• Use 97 per cent fat-free mayonnaise.

Question 14

• Use low-fat mature cheese, low-fat soft cheese like ricotta or cottage and light cream cheese of around 10 per cent fat.

Stay positive and persevere. The changes will soon become old habits!

Fuel of choice for exercise

Before we look at the benefits of exercise, it's appropriate to consider carbohydrates as the fuel of choice for exercising muscles. When we eat carbohydrate, it eventually ends up stored as glycogen in the muscles and the liver. It's then released as needed into the bloodstream as glucose, or blood sugar. Glycogen stores need to be replaced, so it's essential that we regularly eat enough carbohydrate. The amount of carbohydrate we need to eat to replenish our glycogen stores depends largely on the amount of exercise we do. Normally, the body stores enough glycogen to last for 90 minutes of hard exercise. If you are training hard and often feel tired, it may be due to a lack of carbohydrates. You would be well advised to see a dietitian qualified in sports nutrition.

At the same time, it's very important not to *overeat* carbohydrates. That's because glycogen (the principal store of carbohydrates in the body) can be stored only in limited amounts

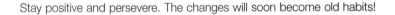

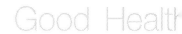

in the liver and the muscles. Once this is exceeded, the extra carbohydrate can be turned into fat and stored in the adipose tissue. In my practice I often see clients who, despite lowering the amount of fats in their diet, still fail to lose weight. The reason: they are still eating too much carbohydrate. If this sounds like you, it may be a good idea to get some help from a qualified nutritionist and check your carbohydrate portions.

You'll find more information on nutrition for athletes by visiting my website: www.nutrition4health.com.au

The benefits of exercise

The human body is a machine designed to move. Our ancestors covered great distances on foot. The invention of the automobile made our feet redundant for covering long distances. Necessity turned into choice, and figures now show that two out of three Australians don't do any exercise. Yet regular exercise has the following benefits:

- Increased physical fitness.
- Increased cardiovascular fitness.
- Weight control or weight loss.
- Regulation of appetite.
- Increased self-esteem.
- Stress release.
- People who exercise regularly may find it easier to give up excessive alcohol consumption or overeating.

Physical fitness has a number of components, all of which are relevant to physical health:

- Cardiovascular fitness.
- Muscular strength and endurance.

- Flexibility.
- Body composition.

Let's look briefly at each of these components.

CARDIOVASCULAR FITNESS

This is the most important component of fitness, the body's aerobic power. It refers to our body's ability to take in oxygen as we breathe and transport it to the exercising muscles to release the fuel that keeps us going. Regular aerobic exercise helps to strengthen the heart and improves our fitness level. The level of cardiovascular fitness can be estimated by measuring our maximal oxygen consumption, or VO_{2max}. The higher our VO_{2max} figure, the better. Elite athletes capable of winning medals at the Olympic Games have staggering figures of around 6 litres per minute, whereas the rest of us fall somewhere between 1.5 and 4 litres per minute. If the closest you come to doing any exercise is watching sport on television, then you may find you are around the bottom end of this scale.

The better your cardiovascular fitness, the less tired you become at a given activity level and the longer you can keep it up. Your cardiovascular fitness can improve with training. If you have been sedentary, you can increase your cardiovascular fitness by 30 per cent by starting an appropriate exercise routine. Your exercise needs to be aerobic—that is, it must increase both your breathing rate and your heart rate.

Estimating your appropriate level of cardiovascular exercise
Beginners. A good workout for beginners brings the heart rate up to 50–60 per cent of the maximum heart rate. The maximum heart rate is an estimate of the highest number of heartbeats, or heart contractions, the heart is capable of in one minute. It differs

between individuals and depends on age. You can calculate your maximum heart rate in the following way:

$$220 - \text{Your age} = \text{Maximum heart rate (MHR)}$$

To work out your desired heart rate per minute during aerobic exercise, multiply your MHR (calculated above) by 0.55 (any-where between 0.50 and 0.60 is fine). Remember this number and compare it to your heart rate while you exercise. It is easy to measure your heart rate by taking your pulse from the carotid artery in the neck. As it's easier to measure your pulse for 15 seconds rather than a full minute, calculate the number of beats you are aiming for per 15 seconds by dividing your desired heart rate per minute by four.

Intermediate level. To further improve your cardiovascular fitness and enhance weight loss, you need to increase your heart rate and maintain it in the range of 60–80 per cent of your MHR. Multiply your MHR (calculated above) by 0.6. This will give you the lower limit for your pulse rate per minute during aerobic exercise of intermediate intensity. For the upper limit of the intermediate level, multiply your MHR by 0.8. This gives you the upper desired rate per minute during any aerobic exercise.

It's best to increase your exercise intensity gradually, over weeks to months, depending on your age, fitness and exercise routine. You may wish to join a gym and work out on equip-ment while wearing a heart monitor, which will show you your heart rate at any given moment. Another way to monitor the increasing intensity of your exercise program is to take your pulse once a week, five minutes into the exercise, for 15 sec-onds, then multiply that number by four to calculate your heartbeats per minute. Compare this figure with your desired heart rate.

2 Case study

Commencing regular exercise

John Smith is a busy IT consultant whose job doesn't involve any physical work. In fact, John spends most of his day sitting in front of his computer. Up to the age of 30 John played competitive football on weekends and worked out in a gym five times a week. Gradually his exercise routine fell apart. Now John can't recall doing any regular exercise for at least six months. He's not particularly worried about his health, but he has noticed that his belt feels somewhat tight lately, and he feels better leaving the top button on his business shirt undone. He does admit that he hasn't got the same amount of energy as he used to have.

During his last visit to his GP, John underwent a regular physical examination, including a weight check. He was dismayed to find that he now weighed around 12 kilograms (26.4 pounds) more than in his fit days. His doctor advised John to take up some regular walking, as this is the most convenient type of exercise and shouldn't take up too much time—a very precious commodity in John's busy life. John found it helpful to consolidate his aims using the following exercise diary.

Age: *43 years*   Maximum heart rate (MHR): *220 − 43 = 177*

Current exercise routine: *I haven't exercised in the last six months.*

Recommended level of aerobic exercise to start with: *Beginner's level.*

John kept records for the first six weeks. He then continued without jotting down his pulse rate, as it became second nature to go out walking and keep up a good aerobic workout. Below is a copy of John's exercise diary.

Aerobic exercise	Week	My pulse rate	% of MHR	My aim
Walking	1	92	0.52	0.55 = 97
	2	97	0.55	0.55 = 97
	3	102	0.58	0.6 = 106
	4	104	0.59	0.6 = 106
	5	110	0.62	0.65 = 115
	6	112	0.63	0.65 = 115

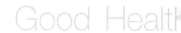

You may wish to keep a similar record to get yourself started. You can download a variety of exercise diaries from my website: www.nutrition4health.com.au

Aerobic exercise progress diary

My weekly exercise routine:

_____ ☐ aerobic

_____ ☐ aerobic

_____ ☐ aerobic

My maximum heart rate is 220 – ____ (age) = ____ beats per minute

Starting date: _____

Aerobic exercise	Week	My pulse rate	% of MHR	My aim
	1			
	2			
	3			
	4			
	5			
	6			
	7			
	8			
	9			
	10			
	11			
	12			
	13			
	14			

The hardest part is *starting* exercising. Once you have started, you will find it easy to keep it up because you will actually feel better! You will have more energy and your body will start to 'remind' you to exercise. Of course, you must have the right workout to suit you. Make sure it's not too hard or too easy. And remember: start gently, and work on improving your fitness gradually.

Exercise will help you stay in shape

Person A ate lunch sitting at the desk and then carried on working.
Person B took a 30-minute walk during the lunch break, and then returned to the office and ate lunch. The exercise burned more calories and caused the metabolic rate to increase, which remained elevated for some time after the walk. As a result, person B burned the food kilojoules consumed at lunch faster than did person A, whose metabolic rate wasn't elevated through exercise. In fact, person B could eat around 10 per cent more kilojoules than person A and still maintain weight on that day.

MUSCULAR STRENGTH AND ENDURANCE, AND FLEXIBILITY

Adequate levels of strength, muscular endurance (stamina) and flexibility are important for living an active and independent life. What levels are considered adequate will vary from person to person. Good abdominal strength/endurance and hip flexibility are important for good posture, an enhanced sex life, and the prevention of muscular and skeletal injuries.

Good exercises for improving strength are weightlifting with light weights, and circuit classes; and for flexibility try yoga, tai chi, or just gentle flexing exercises done at home on a regular basis.

BODY COMPOSITION

Bone, muscle and adipose tissue are the main components of our body's weight. A person's weight measurement alone does not differentiate between these components. Although for most people an accurate scale is sufficient to measure weight changes, which represent mostly fat loss, in athletes this may be rather crude. In athletes, fat loss, accompanied by bulking up of muscles, is determined more accurately by measuring body fat using skinfold calipers. It's impossible to do a skinfold test on yourself; you will need to consult a sports dietitian or a physical trainer if you wish to have your body fat measured. The results are given as a percentage of your body weight. It may be useful to track your body fat levels over a period of time if you are training to compete in athletic events that require low body fat levels, such as running and cycling.

Aim to keep your weight within a healthy range

- Surplus fat slows down physical performance in many sport disciplines.
- Excessive body fat predisposes to late onset diabetes, high blood pressure and heart disease.
- Too little fat predisposes to increased susceptibility to illness, fatigue, and irregular periods or lack of periods in women.

For most people, keeping their weight within the healthy weight range (check your weight against your height in the chart below), maintains a healthy amount of body fat. If you don't exercise, you may need a bit of muscle toning. You can burn fat and build up muscle tone by increasing your aerobic exercise to three times a week for at least half an hour each session.

Weight for height chart for men and women aged 18–64

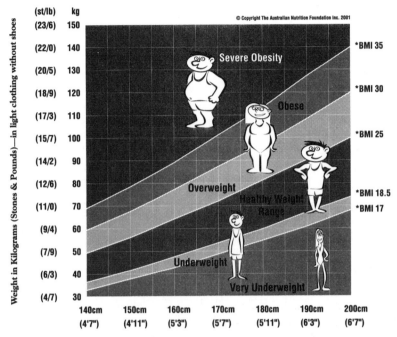

Aim for the Healthy Weight Range

© Copyright The Australian Nutrition Foundation Inc. 2001

Weight in Kilograms (Stones & Pounds)—in light clothing without shoes

Severe Obesity

Obese

Overweight

Healthy Weight Range

Underweight

Very Underweight

*BMI 35

*BMI 30

*BMI 25

*BMI 18.5

*BMI 17

(st/lb)	kg
(23/6)	150
(22/0)	140
(20/5)	130
(18/9)	120
(17/3)	110
(15/7)	100
(14/2)	90
(12/6)	80
(11/0)	70
(9/4)	60
(7/9)	50
(6/3)	40
(4/7)	30

140cm (4'7")   150cm (4'11")   160cm (5'3")   170cm (5'7")   180cm (5'11")   190cm (6'3")   200cm (6'7")

Height in Centimetres (Feet & Inches)—without shoes

* Body Mass Index (BMI) = $\dfrac{\text{Weight (kg)}}{\text{Height}^2 \text{ (metres)}}$

Optimal health through food variety and physical activity

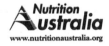

A Nutrition Australia
www.nutritionaustralia.org

Let's look at your exercise routine

checkpoint **5**

	Yes	No
1. Do you exercise at least three times a week?	☐	☐
2. Do you exercise for at least 30 minutes, three times a week, using any of the following methods?		
Walking	☐	☐
Running	☐	☐
Cycling	☐	☐
Swimming	☐	☐
Aerobics	☐	☐
Circuit classes	☐	☐
Rowing	☐	☐

3. Do you include any of the following in your
   exercise routine?
   Yoga   ☐   ☐
   Tai chi   ☐   ☐
   Other stretching/flexing exercises   ☐   ☐
4. Do you include weightlifting in your
   exercise routine?   ☐   ☐

✔ If you answered 'Yes' at least once to all four questions in Checkpoint 4, you have a balanced exercise routine that will keep you fit, improve your muscle tone and keep you flexible—congratulations!

✗ If you answered 'No' to the first question, increase your exercise to at least three times weekly to get significantly more benefit.

✗ If you answered 'No' to the second question, your cardiovascular fitness is compromised. This is the most important component for most of us. Work on improving your cardiovascular fitness. Make a commitment to start exercising and aim to do three 30-minute aerobic exercise sessions a week. Choose any activity from the list in question 2 above. Walking is probably the most convenient, and certainly the cheapest, form of aerobic exercise.

✗ If you answered 'No' to the third question, you might consider taking up yoga or including some stretches as part of your daily routine. Five minutes in the morning is a good start.

✗ If you answered 'No' to the last question, you might consider combining some gentle weightlifting with your aerobic exercise to increase your muscular strength and/or muscle tone.

You may wish to consult a personal trainer to work out a suitable exercise routine for you.

The waist-to-hip ratio—the shape as well as weight

Where our body stores its excess fat is very important. Scientists now know that some people are at a higher risk than others for chronic diseases such as diabetes, depending on where they carry any extra fat. There are two possibilities: on the trunk or the upper body, and on the hips or the lower body. The two body types are referred to as *apple* and *pear* shapes, respectively.

Be aware of any health limitations before starting an exercise routine. If you are excessively overweight, suffer from high blood pressure or are convalescing from a leg joint injury, talk to your doctor before starting.

Characteristics of an apple-shaped body are small hips in proportion to the waist, and a tummy pouch on side view. Characteristics of a pear-shaped body are a thin waist, wider hips and a thin upper body. Men store excess weight in apple shapes. Women can be either shape.

If you are carrying excess weight, carrying it on the tummy (apple shape) places you at a higher risk for heart disease, diabetes and high blood pressure. This type of excess weight is called android obesity. Where excess weight is carried on the hips (pear shape), it's called gynecoid obesity. The waist-to-hip ratio is a simple measurement that allows you to work out which model you fit into. To work out your waist-to-hip ratio, take your hip and waist measurements in centimetres. Take the measurements three times and then work out the averages for your hips and waist. Then divide your average waist measurement by your average hip measurement. If you are a woman and your waist-to-hip ratio is above 0.8, you are an apple shape (less is pear shape). For men an apple shape corresponds to a ratio of 0.95 and above. The box below provides an example.

Calculating the waist-to-hip ratio

Molly has the following measurements:
Waist average: 75 cm (29.5 inches)
Hip average: 102 cm (40.2 inches)
Her waist-to-hip ratio is: 75 divided by 102 = 0.74
Molly therefore has a pear-shaped figure.

What does the waist-to-hip result tell us? If your waist-to-hip ratio is less than 0.8 (for a woman) or 0.95 (for a man), then you are less likely to suffer from chronic diseases associated with being overweight. If it is higher than 0.8 (for a woman) or 0.95 (for a man), then you are more likely to suffer from heart disease, diabetes and high blood pressure. You are also particularly prone to developing diabetes and heart disease if your waist measurement at the level of your navel is more than 90 cm (35.43 inches) for women and 100 cm (39.37 inches) for men. In simpler terms, if you store your excess energy in an apple shape, then you are more likely to suffer from these conditions than a pear-shaped person of the same weight and gender. It's therefore especially important for you to reduce your weight!

chapter five

Nutrition and heart health

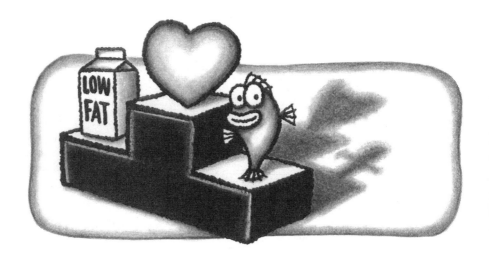

■ GOALS

- To reduce the amount of saturated fat in your diet
- To consume no more than 30 per cent of your total kilojoules in the form of fats
- To limit cholesterol-rich foods
- To increase omega-3 fatty acids in your diet
- To increase antioxidants in your diet

■ BENEFITS

- You will reduce the risk of developing heart disease
- You will enjoy a healthier, more fruitful life for longer

It's often difficult to understand the value of benefits that are not felt immediately. This is particularly true in the case of heart disease—after all, we don't feel any different regardless of what our cholesterol level is. It may be helpful to use an analogy when talking about the benefits of looking after your heart. When we take out life insurance, we don't experience the benefits of the insurance immediately, and yet many people still choose to take out life insurance because they accept the possibility of accidental death. In the same way, we may not experience the immediate benefits of looking after our heart, but we will be thankful later when the 'premiums' we have paid by looking after our health early on pay off in a longer, healthier life.

Four out of ten people will die of heart disease. It's the biggest cause of premature death in the Western world. A balanced diet is an important player in preventing premature death from heart disease. It's one of the best ways to ensure you will not suffer from heart disease.

Atherosclerosis

The heart is a strong muscle which, when it contracts, pumps blood to every part of the body. Its regular rhythm is set in motion in our early development as an unborn baby and continues until our death. Premature death due to heart disease is the major cause of early death in adults in Australia.

Chronic damage to the arteries—the blood vessels that carry oxygenated blood to our muscles and tissues, including the heart—is called atherosclerosis. In approximately 98 per cent of people, atherosclerosis is caused by poor lifestyle habits, with poor diet being a key contributing factor. Only around 2 per cent of the general population have a strong inherited predisposition to develop heart disease, usually diagnosed in childhood. Diet and other lifestyle factors remain important, in addition to medication, in genetically induced heart disease.

Heart disease is not a disease of old age, although the risk of suffering from heart disease increases with age. People die of heart disease as early as in their thirties and forties. You probably know someone who is middle-aged, perhaps a relative or neighbour, who is now following a strict low-fat diet and walking every day after surviving a heart attack. The majority of people who survive a heart attack develop an enormous resolve to follow any guideline, no matter how strict, in order to avoid repeating the experience. Having counselled people who have had open-heart surgery, I know that rehabilitation isn't fun. It's far easier, and a lot cheaper, to prevent heart disease occurring than to cure it.

Check your risk profile for heart disease by completing the quiz in Checkpoint 6.

Checking your risk profile for heart disease

checkpoint **6**

Take a minute to read through the following lists. Circle the crosses or ticks that apply to you. Circle '?' if you are unsure.

INCREASED RISK	LOWER RISK
✘ Raised cholesterol level	✔ Low saturated fat diet
✘ Raised triglyceride levels	?
✘ Smoking	✔ Adequate antioxidant intake
✘ High blood pressure	?
✘ Diabetes	✔ Healthy weight
✘ Lack of exercise	?
✘ Being overweight	✔ Regular aerobic exercise
✘ Stress—type A personality	?

Your score: *Number of crosses:* ____   *Number of ticks:* ____

Did you have any crosses? The higher the number of crosses, the higher your chances of developing heart disease. Aim to pick up all of the positive habits next to the ticks. If you weren't sure and circled the question marks, then read on to find the answers.

Understanding heart disease

It was the renowned Italian physician Leonardo da Vinci who had the first glimpse of atherosclerosis. In the sixteenth century Leonardo da Vinci performed illegal, detailed autopsies on the heart and the arteries without as yet being aware of the body's circulatory system. During one of his dissections he came across what appeared to be lumps on the inside of a blood vessel. Upon further inspection he described them as being like orange rind. He was looking at what we now call plaque, a deposit of dead cells, cholesterol and other organic waste. Once formed, plaque obstructs the circulation of blood around the body. We can't feel the plaque forming; however, if left unchecked, given time it will lead to pain as heart disease sets in.

Having a high cholesterol level increases your chances of developing atherosclerosis.

ANGINA

'I have recurring pain on the left side where my heart is. I get it when I walk uphill, or if the dog takes me for a little run in the morning. I'm sure it's nothing, but I just though I'd mention it.'

What this person is describing is the classic symptoms of angina, a sign that the circulation to the heart muscle is faulty. Due to a partial blockage of the artery caused by plaque, not enough oxygenated blood is reaching the heart, and the result is severe pain. Angina is usually, but not always, felt during physical activity when the heart needs to beat faster to meet the additional demands for oxygen of the exercising muscles.

If you ever experience this type of pain, bring it to the attention of your doctor at once. Angina is a warning that shouldn't be ignored. The degree of blockage in your arteries must be assessed and treated medically.

HEART ATTACK

If the blockage in the artery leading to the heart muscle is severe enough to significantly block the blood flow to the heart, it will cause the heart to stop altogether. The symptoms of a heart attack are described as an extreme squeezing pain around the breastbone, sometimes travelling to the back or down the left arm. This is a very painful experience and can be fatal.

SURGICAL TREATMENT OF HEART DISEASE

One form of surgical treatment is coronary angioplasty, also known as balloon treatment. A small balloon is inserted into the artery wall through a tube and is then inflated. The inflated balloon flattens the cholesterol plaque against the artery wall, restoring blood flow to the heart.

In a coronary artery bypass, a vein or small artery usually from the leg is grafted on to the damaged artery so as to bypass it. The bypass then detours the blood flow around the blockage.

Both of these surgical procedures may require long periods of convalescence. Neither procedure is foolproof. Without lifestyle modification plaque build-up will continue, and there is strong evidence that it will proceed at a faster rate. Diet and other lifestyle factors therefore become even more important in helping to prevent ongoing damage to the arteries and avoiding another heart attack.

Blood cholesterol

Cholesterol is a fat-derived, waxy substance that our bodies make naturally. It is also present in many foods we eat. Cholesterol can become a problem if its levels in the blood rise too high.

CHOLESTEROL TESTS

Although we can't feel the gradual build-up of plaque, testing our cholesterol level is one way of keeping an eye on the health of our arteries. Cholesterol is measured through a simple blood test. If you are over 30 and haven't yet had your cholesterol levels tested, see your doctor to arrange a test.

The results are presented as different fractions or types of cholesterol: LDL cholesterol and HDL cholesterol. LDL cholesterol is like a barge filled to the brim with Edam cheese that is about to capsize and spill its contents. HDL cholesterol is like a coastguard on the lookout for any sinking barges. HDL cholesterol gives protection against the build-up of plaque by preventing the LDL cholesterol from 'capsizing' and depositing itself in the artery wall.

USA recommendations
Total cholesterol <200 mg/dl
HDL ≥35 mg/dl

In a nutshell

- LDL cholesterol—harmful if too high.
- HDL cholesterol—the higher it is, the better protection it provides against plaque deposits.

Here are some figures against which you can check your own test results. In Australia, the National Heart Foundation recommends testing cholesterol levels every five years if there is no family history of heart disease, and if no previous test, including the latest one, gave a result higher than 5.5 mmol/l. If your result is above 5.5 mmol/l, then you must see your doctor regarding treatment. If it is above 6.5 mmol/l, you should be tested again after three months. It's not necessary to fast before the initial test, as total cholesterol levels are not substantially increased by a recent meal. Aim to keep your LDL cholesterol below 3.5 mmol/l and your HDL cholesterol above 1 mmol/l.

European recommendations
Total cholesterol <5 mmol/l
LDL cholesterol <3.0 mmol/l
HDL cholesterol >1.0 mmol/l

THE RATIO OF TOTAL CHOLESTEROL TO HDL CHOLESTEROL

The ratio of total cholesterol to HDL cholesterol helps to assess the current risk of heart disease. Statistically, the average risk falls between 3.5 and 4.5. If your ratio falls above 4.5, you have an increased risk of suffering from atherosclerosis. You would be advised by your doctor to change any lifestyle habits that increase your likelihood of developing this heart disease, and to commence medication if your risk is particularly high. The higher the ratio, the higher the risk of heart disease.

CHOLESTEROL-LOWERING MEDICATION

Medication is necessary for some people who are unable to lower their cholesterol levels by following a suitable diet and exercise program alone. However, if you were considering using medication as the first and only treatment, keep in mind that it is not a cure-all and may have side effects.

Common drugs used to lower cholesterol levels

HMG Co-A reductase inhibitors ('statins'): Long-term safety not well demonstrated.

Bile acid resins (e.g. cholestyramine): Not altogether well tolerated.

Fibric acid-based medication (e.g. gemfibrozil): Not always effective in lowering cholesterol.

Nicotinic acid: Not well tolerated.

Probucol: Has an uncertain role in therapy.

Source: Consensus Cholesterol and Cardiovascular Health: A Practical Approach: an interactive education programme for general practitioners on the management of hyper lipidaemia: moderators guide, Sydney: Oxford Clinical Communications Australia, 1992

If your doctor has placed you on cholesterol-lowering medication, *don't discontinue or change your medication by yourself.* Always talk to your doctor. Do consider diet modification if you have not already done so.

DIET VERSUS MEDICATION

A healthy diet can make a difference and should be the first therapy you undertake to reduce a high cholesterol level if you have no family history of heart disease or other risk factors. Only consider using medication if your cholesterol level still remains high after at least six weeks of diet therapy. Ideally, diet therapy should be trialled for six months.

If the risk for heart disease is particularly high, then cholesterol medication together with a suitable diet may be needed. Follow your doctor's advice, based on your individual needs. Taking cholesterol medication while continuing to eat a high-fat diet is like keeping a guard dog in the backyard and leaving the front door open on your way out. It's not a wise way to guard your heart's health. Finding the cause of elevated cholesterol and correcting it is the only real long-term solution. Which brings us to your eating habits.

Optimum nutrition for heart health

There is an immense variety of foods available for our consumption today. Each food is made up of a myriad of chemicals. When we digest and absorb food, these food chemicals become short- or long-lasting body chemicals. Food ingredients become chemicals transported in our bloodstream. What is transported, and how much, is a direct reflection of our diet. Diet is the source not only of all the nutrients but also of the wastes and excesses that find their way into the body's circulatory system.

Thus, there is no doubt that diet influences the health of the heart. Positive changes to your diet will prevent further damage to your heart and circulation, and there is good evidence that it may reverse some of the damage already done.

Let's now look at the key players in our diet that influence heart health, and what changes are beneficial to our heart health.

SATURATED FATS

Saturated fats increase LDL cholesterol. Keep them to a minimum in your diet. Saturated fats are found in both animal and vegetable foods. However, in the typical Western diet, the majority of saturated fat comes from animal fats. You will spot saturated fats easily if you remember that they are solid at room temperature.

Sources of saturated fats

Animal sources
- Dairy foods (milk fat) e.g. butter
- Lard, tallow, suet
- Meat fat, poultry fat

Plant sources
- Copha, hydrogenated table margarine
- Palm oil, palm kernel oil
- Coconut oil, coconut cream and coconut milk
- Blended vegetable oils—blends of coconut or palm kernel oil. These oils are used widely in the manufacture of cakes, biscuits and some ready-made meals.

For a supermarket tour showing food products high in saturated fat and suitable alternatives, visit www.nutrition4health.com.au

Practical hints for keeping a lid on saturated fats

✓ Cut out saturated fat items that you eat out of habit and find alternatives you will enjoy eating.

✓ Keep your favourite high-fat foods for special occasions.

✓ Eat a smaller portion of foods containing a lot of saturated fats (e.g. appetiser size not main meal size).

You may want to consult with a dietitian to help you make the necessary changes to your diet. However, this chapter contains a lot of useful information and handy hints. You may feel that you are on the right track after you have finished reading.

Reading ingredient lists

Labelling laws may not require the manufacturers of food items to specify fats in terms of whether they are saturated, monounsaturated or polyunsaturated; they are only required to indicate whether they are vegetable or animal fats. As vegetable fats can be saturated as well as unsaturated, it is best to assume that it is saturated and avoid it in the interests of your heart's health.

Coconut oil is a relatively cheap fat and is used widely in processed foods. So, keep an eye out for 'vegetable oil' when reading ingredient lists; it's probably coconut fat.

Avoid buying foods that are high in saturated fats, and don't forget to look at the overall fat content. Aim for a ceiling of 10 per cent.

TRANS FATTY ACIDS

Trans fatty acids form during the process of fat hydrogenation or solidifying, such as during the manufacture of margarine from oils. The evidence suggests that they act similarly to saturated fats and raise blood cholesterol levels; therefore, you should aim to minimise your consumption of these acids. The percentage of trans fatty acids in margarines varies between 8 and 10 per cent. Butter has 5 per cent trans fatty acids.

To reduce the amount of trans fatty acids in your diet, avoid regular hydrogenated margarines and hydrogenated oils. Always check ingredient lists for these. Some spreads are available on the market with as little as 0.4–0.6 per cent trans fatty acids.

DIETARY CHOLESTEROL

Dietary cholesterol eaten in excess raises blood cholesterol. Avoid eating foods that are extremely high in cholesterol. Aim for a cholesterol intake of below 300 milligrams if you are at a high risk of heart disease. Cholesterol is found only in foods of animal origin. There is no cholesterol in plant foods.

The following foods are rich sources of cholesterol and are best avoided or limited:

- offal
- brains
- tripe
- lamb's fry
- paté
- fish roe
- egg yolks

New spreads on the market

You have probably seen spreads enriched with plant sterols in the supermarket by now. Plant sterols occur naturally in most plant foods in amounts of about half a gram per kilogram. Research on these substances shows that they lower LDL cholesterol (the 'bad' type of cholesterol) by up to 15 per cent. They do so by lowering the absorption of cholesterol from our intestine. The recommended amount of plant sterols to achieve this effect is 2–3 grams (0.07–0.102) daily. This translates to eating about four or five teaspoons of the spreads each day.

Remember that the beneficial effect of consuming plant sterols should be complementary to healthy eating habits. If you do have a high cholesterol level, then my recommendation is to use these spreads in place of butter or other margarines, and not in excess of four teaspoons daily. The spreads are best used for spreading or in baking. Avoid overheating as extreme heat—frying, for example—will change their beneficial properties, and affect the taste.

I recommend eating yellow fruits and vegetables each day to keep up a good amount of carotenoids in your diet, as some studies have shown that the absorption of carotenoids is lowered if plant sterols-enriched spreads are consumed in the recommended amounts.

Seafood and cholesterol

The fruits of the sea (oysters, mussels, squid, prawns, Balmain bugs, and so on) are low in saturated fat, total fat and (with the exception of squid, prawns, lobster and fish roe) cholesterol. The good news is that the cholesterol in seafood doesn't contribute significantly to our blood cholesterol level. It's far more important to reduce *saturated* fat, and in most cases total fat, than to limit low-fat foods that are high in cholesterol. Because squid, lobster, prawns and fish roe are very low in saturated and total fats, we can include them in our diets. If you have a very high cholesterol level, enjoy them in moderation—say, once or twice a week. Just keep them away from the deep-fryer!

TRIGLYCERIDES

Triglyceride is a scientific name for food fat once it has found its way into our bloodstream. Too much saturated fat, alcohol or sugar can increase triglyceride levels. A high triglyceride level increases the risk of heart disease. Balance out your diet to prevent excessive triglycerides.

To keep your triglycerides in check:

- Avoid eating too much fat—you can work out a healthy level for yourself using the information on the following pages.
- Keep your weight within the healthy weight range.
- Enjoy alcohol in moderation.
- Cut down on sugar or sweets if you are overweight.

Fat

A high-fat diet predisposes to weight gain. Weight gain is usually accompanied by increased cholesterol levels, blood pressure and increases the chance of developing diabetes. Avoid eating too much fat.

If you are overweight, reduce all types of fats in your diet so as to reduce your weight to within the healthy weight range for your height.

HOW MUCH FAT IS RECOMMENDED?

It's easy to have too much fat in our diet, and this isn't good for us in the long run. At the same time, cutting out *all* fats from the foods we eat can be just as dangerous. So, just how much fat is a good amount? To answer this question, work out your individual healthy daily allowance. The recommended intake of fats is based on your daily energy needs, according to the following guidelines. Here the kilojoule is used as the unit of energy.

- Maximum 10 per cent of kilojoules should come from saturated fats.
- 10–15 per cent of kilojoules should come from monounsaturated fat.
- Maximum 10 per cent of kilojoules should come from polyunsaturated fat.

In practice, for women with an average activity level (needing 7560 kilojoules or 1800 calories daily) this works out to be about a tablespoon of each type of fat daily. For men with an average activity level (needing 10 080 kilojoules or 2400 calories daily) this works out to be about a tablespoon and a half of each type of fat.

How much fat do you use in food preparation, and how does this compare with the amounts recommended above? If you are using butter, a saturated fat, to spread on your toast and bread and you have gone through a tablespoon of butter by breakfast, you are definitely overdoing it!

Work out your optimum daily fat amount

- *Step 1:* Write down your daily energy needs in kilojoules (refer back to the 'Calculating your average daily energy needs' box in Chapter 4): .
- *Step 2:* Multiply the figure from step 1 by three and then divide by ten. This gives you the recommended amount of energy in kilojoules to be supplied by fats in your diet.
- *Step 3:* Divide the figure from step 2 by 37. This gives you the recommended amount of fat in grams. Remember this figure.

The healthy amount of fat for me is ____ grams a day.

To change grams into tablespoons, divide by 20. To change grams into teaspoons, divide by five. To convert grams to ounces divide by 28.3.

Turn to the table called 'Hidden fats in the foods we eat' on p. 82 and compare your figure to the amount of fat present in some common foods. *Remember: your figure is the total recommended fat intake in grams for the day, regardless of whether it is added to or present as part of a food.*

Mark decides to lower his cholesterol level

Mark decided to see a dietitian to help reduce his cholesterol level. In addition to lowering his saturated fat intake, he has been advised to lower his total fat intake to lower his body weight, which is 6 kilograms (13.2 pounds) above the upper figure of his healthy weight range. The dietitian asked Mark to keep a record of what he ate and drank for a week to determine his average daily fat intake. Here is one day's entries, together with the fat intake as calculated by the dietitian.

MEAL	FOOD AND DRINK	FAT IN GRAMS
Breakfast	½ cup toasted muesli	9 (¼ oz)
	Glass regular milk	8 (¼ oz)
	Orange juice	0
Snack	3 choc-chip biscuits	10 (⅓ oz)
	Coffee, black	0
Lunch	2 cheese sandwiches	20 (⅔ oz)
	2 teaspoons margarine	10 (⅓ oz)
	Apple	0
	Diet Coke	0
Snack	Banana	0
Dinner	200 g steak	20 (⅔ oz)
	Steamed vegetables	0
	Mashed potato	5 (⅙ oz)
	Mineral water	0
	TOTAL = 82 g	

Mark's daily energy needs are 8820 kilojoules (1950 calories), and the recommended amount from fat is 2900 kilojoules (690 calories), or 70 grams

(2½ oz) of fat. Mark's total daily fat intake was 82 grams (2⅘ oz), so on that day he exceeded the recommended fat intake by 12 grams (⅖ oz).

The dietitian made a few suggestions, including:

✓ Switching over to a lower-fat milk.

✓ Eating untoasted muesli.

✓ Using fat-reduced cheddar cheese.

These suggestions alone lowered Mark's fat intake by 4, 4 and 5 (⅐, ⅐ and ⅙ oz): total 13 grams (½ oz) respectively. This reduced Mark's fat intake to 69 grams (2⅖ oz)—within the recommended healthy limit. In addition, Mark decided to omit margarine when preparing sandwiches. This saved him a further 10 grams (⅓ oz) of fat. His new total of 59 grams (2 oz) daily represents 25 per cent of his total energy needs.

Mark's dietitian also suggested limiting sugar and increasing aerobic exercise. Combined with his new daily fat intake, this would allow Mark to lose half a kilogram (approximately 1 pound) of surplus body fat a week. It will take him 12 weeks (three months) to lose 6 kilograms (1 stone) and get down to a healthy weight. Three months is also a good time to test his cholesterol level again. By lowering his weight and his saturated fat intake, Mark's cholesterol level should follow suit.

You may like to visit my website www.nutrition4health.com.au where you can receive individual feedback on the amount of fat in your diet.

SETTING UP A 'FAT ACCOUNT'

A 'fat account' is a credit account where instead of balancing out money, you balance out fat grams. Imagine a figure in your fat account that is your opening account balance; you can draw from it at your leisure providing you don't exceed the limit. While in the real world if you don't keep within your budget you will be penalised with a steep interest rate by your bank, if you don't keep to your fat limit you will be penalised by weight gain, and possibly a significant rise in cholesterol levels.

Your account is set at X grams of fat daily, depending on your sex, weight, height, and so on. (If you worked out your optimum daily fat amount this is your daily opening balance figure.) This figure remains constant from day to day. Each time you eat in excess of your daily fat figure you go into overdraft. If you continually overeat or borrow it will catch up with you eventually. Instead of a steep interest charge, however, you will be paying with your health. And we all know that health is more precious than gold!

How John can balance his fat account

4 Case study

John is a busy accountant who often works long hours. He is working late today and decides he will drop into a local café for a snack at around 5 p.m. to keep up his energy level. He chooses cheesecake and coffee and, as an afterthought, an apple, as his wife pointed out recently that he's not looking after his diet.

Let's have a look at the fat grams in John's snack:

Cheesecake	36 grams	(1¼ oz)
Apple	0 grams	(0 oz)
Coffee, long black	0 grams	(0 oz)
Total fat grams	36 grams	(1¼ oz)
John's daily opening balance	76 grams	(2⅔ oz)

By eating the cheesecake, John has used up approximately half of his daily fat allowance. Even if he had avoided eating a fatty breakfast and lunch, John's dinner must be low in fat for him to stay within his fat budget for the day. Good choices that would enable him to stay within his fat budget would be grilled, steamed or baked (without added fat) lean meat, chicken or fish, with vegetables cooked by any of these methods. He

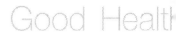

would have to avoid fatty sauces or oily salad dressings. He could use a variety of low-fat sauces or low-fat gravy.

You don't have to become a guru on the fat content of foods. This, together with other food analysis, is the job of a nutritionist. But it does help in your quest to keep within your fat account balance if you are familiar with some everyday foods and their lower-fat alternatives.

Hidden fats in the foods we eat

BREADS AND CEREALS	FAT (approximately)	
Garlic bread (2 slices)	12 g	(²/₅ oz)
Bread (2 slices)	1 g	(negligible)
Toasted muesli (½ cup)	9 g	(⅓ oz)
Breakfast cereal (average bowl)	1 g	(negligible)
DAIRY PRODUCTS		
Regular milk 1 cup	8 g	(¼ oz)
Reduced-fat milk 1 cup	3 g	(¹/₁₀ oz)
Skim milk 1 cup	0 g	—
Mature cheese (1 slice)	8 g	(¼ oz)
Cottage cheese ½ cup	2 g	(¹/₁₄ oz)
Yoghurt, regular 1 tub	9 g	(⅓ oz)
Yoghurt, non-fat 1 tub	<1 g	(negligible)
Cream (1 tblspn)	8 g	(¼ oz)
Ice-cream (2 scoops)	6 g	(⅕ oz)
Ice-cream, rich (2 small scoops)	13 g	(??? oz)
MEATS		
Chicken (2 drumsticks with skin)	15 g	(½ oz)

Chicken breast fillet	2 g	(1/14 oz)
Steak (150 g or 5⅓ oz, trimmed, grilled)	10 g	(⅓ oz)
Lamb loin chops (2 grilled)	32 g	(1 oz)
Lamb leg roast (85 g, trimmed)	6 g	(⅕ oz)
Pork leg steak (120 g, grilled)	4 g	(1/7 oz)
Veal schnitzel (150 g)	14 g	(½ oz)
Sausages (2 grilled)	30 g	(1 oz)

FAST FOODS

Hamburger (1 large)	30 g	(1 oz)
BBQ chicken (quarter)	15 g	(½ oz)
Meat pie/sausage roll	24 g	(⅘ oz)
Pizza, thin crust (quarter)	15 g	(½ oz)
Chinese meal (average serve)	16 g	(½ oz)
Fish in batter	24 g	(⅘ oz)

CAKES, BISCUITS AND SNACKS

Chocolate cake (average slice)	15 g	(½ oz)
Cheesecake (average slice)	36 g	(1¼ oz)
Apple pie (average slice)	19 g	(⅔ oz)
Croissant	15 g	(½ oz)
Chocolate-coated biscuits (2)	7 g	(⅕ oz)
Potato crisps (small packet)	16 g	(½ oz)
Nuts (50 g)	23 g	(⅘ oz)
Chocolate (100 g)	27 g	(1 oz)
Muesli bar (fruit)	5 g	(⅙ oz)

SPREADS AND DRESSINGS

Salad dressing (1 tblspn)	16 g	(½ oz)
Mayonnaise (1 tblspn)	16 g	(½ oz)
Avocado (½ medium)	21 g	(⅔ oz)
Oil (1 tblspn)	20 g	(⅔ oz)
Butter/margarine (1 tblspn)	16 g	(½ oz)

Although we have looked at the issue of fats in some detail, I wouldn't expect you to count fat grams on a regular basis. Rather, you can do this occasionally to check the quality of your diet, and I hope this chapter has helped you form a reasonable idea of what your diet is like. If your diet needs a little more work, don't hesitate to contact a qualified nutritionist in your area. This is especially important if, for medical reasons, you must follow a low-fat diet. Finally, I hope this section has given you an incentive for budgeting for your health, targeting fats as one of the most influential players in our diet. Following is a food selection tour through the different food groups. All are well within your fat budget—enjoy!

A guide to selecting low-fat foods

To avoid overeating fat, choose mostly the following foods from each of the food groups.

Meat and alternatives

- Fish and seafood
- Skinless poultry
- Lean/trimmed white meats
- Lean/trimmed red meats
- Lean, unprocessed cold cuts (e.g. ham deluxe, shaved chicken)
- Lentils, dried peas and beans

Dairy products

- Low-fat and fat-reduced dairy products
- Fat-reduced soy products
- Cottage cheese, ricotta cheese, and fat-reduced or low-fat mature cheeses

Cereals and grains

- Breads, rolls, bagels, English muffins, crumpets
- Steamed/boiled rice, pasta
- Wholegrain or wholemeal cereals (untoasted)
- Buckwheat, millet, couscous, barley

Fruit and vegetables

- All fresh fruits
- All fresh vegetables, except avocado and olives (these may be enjoyed in moderation)

Sweets

- Plain biscuits, Turkish delight, jellies, jelly babies, 97 per cent fat-free licorice, 97 per cent fat-free fruit bars (all in moderation)

Essential fats

There are two fats that escape the body's manufacturing skills. They are essential for health, and heart health in particular. These two fats are linoleic and alpha-linolenic acids. They are essential raw materials for the manufacture of many other fatty acids in the body. Let's take a brief look at these fatty acids.

Linoleic acid (w-6 fat)
- gamma-linolenic acid (GLA)—found in primrose oil
  - arachidonic acid (AA)—found in meat
    - numerous w-6 fatty acids

Alpha-linolenic acid (w-3 fat)
- eicosapentaenoic acid *(EPA) found in fish*
  - decosahexaenoic acid *(DHA) found in fish*
    - numerous w-3 fatty acids

FISH OILS

Cold water regions include the waters surrounding North America and northern Europe, in particular Scandinavia. It's these cold waters that maintain the life of herring, sardines, mackerel and other cold-water fish. Europeans eat more cold-water fish than people in Australia or the United States. Herring is probably the most popular, and every menu in Denmark, Sweden, Holland and Germany includes at least one herring dish. It's eaten raw, dried and pickled, and is canned, smoked and exported. You can even get vintage dried herring—a little like the hundred-year-old egg in Chinese cuisine.

It's a worrying statistic that a typical Western diet is very poor in fish. This is despite the availability of a wonderful variety of fish around the world.

So, what is the connection between cold-water fish and heart disease? The amount of w-3 essential fatty acids in cold-water fish is what gives them their nutritional advantage. For example, herring contains good amounts of the w-3 fatty acids eicosapentaenoic acid (EPA) and docosahexaenoic acid (DHA). The levels of EPA and DHA are extremely low in land animals and in plants. They can be made from alpha-linolenic acid, which is found in green leafy vegetables, seeds and nuts, but it takes 10 grams (⅓ oz) of alpha-linolenic acid to make 1 gram (⅟₃₀ oz) of fish oils. In practice this is very uneconomical, and is not a practical way of obtaining these fatty acids from the diet.

OILS AIN'T OILS AND FISH OILS ARE UNIQUE

Due to their unique chemistry, fish oils play an important part in altering blood viscosity. They help to keep the blood from being too sticky, from clotting unnecessarily—something that occurs if there is damage to the insides of our arteries. A clot may bring on a heart attack, as it completes the blockage in an artery that is already partly blocked. Research shows that fish

A typical Western diet, for instance, the Australian diet, is very low in w-3 essential fats, found in cold-water fish such as herring, sardines and mackerel.

eaters have a 70 per cent less chance of suffering a heart attack. Eating fish has the following benefits for your heart:

- It has an anti-thrombotic action—that is, it prevents blood particles sticking together.
- It prevents heart spasms and regulates the heartbeat.
- It prevents vasoconstriction, or narrowing of the arteries.

One study found that 3 grams (1/10 oz) of w-3 fatty acids a day lowered blood fats (triglycerides) by one third. Three grams of w-3 fatty acids is equivalent to 250 grams (8¾ oz) of salmon, 10–12 MaxEPA capsules or four teaspoons of cod liver oil. Fish oils worked as well as Gemfibrozil (the most common drug used to reduce triglycerides) without its side effects! Even one fish meal a day was sufficient to see a significant effect.

Fish-eating eskimos have reduced risk of heart disease

Alaska's Eskimos (or Inuit) top the list for the highest w-3 fatty acid consumption. Their diet is based on fish, seal and whale, all of which are excellent sources of w-3 fatty acids. The levels of w-3 fatty acids are about seven to 13 times higher in Eskimos than in non-native people in Alaska. The rate of heart disease is much lower among Eskimos when compared to non-native Alaskans who eat a mixed Western diet with small amounts of fish.

Sally works out her fish oil needs

5 Case study

Sally suffers from mild angina. Her father died of a heart attack when he was in his sixties. Sally was recently advised to include more fish rich in w-3 fatty acids in her diet. She decided to see a nutritionist to get some practical guidelines. The nutritionist showed Sally how to work out her daily w-3 fatty acid intake and then translated that into food choices. Here are the steps the nutritionist followed.

Step 1: She worked out Sally's daily energy requirement, which was 7560 kilojoules (1800 calories).

Step 2: She multiplied Sally's daily energy needs by 0.3 and again by 0.04. The fraction of w-3 fatty acids should make up 4 per cent of the energy to be supplied by total fats: 7560 X 0.3 X 0.04 = 91 kilojoules (22 calories).

Step 3: Finally, to work out Sally's w-3 fatty acid intake in grams, she divided 91 kilojoules by 37 (1 gram of fat has 37 kilojoules): 91 ÷ 37 = 2.4 grams of w-3 fatty acids.

The daily recommended intake of w-3 fatty acids is given as a range between 4 and 6 per cent of the total recommended daily fat intake. For Sally, 2.4 grams is the lowest recommended intake, while 3.6 grams is the upper limit. Now that she knows her daily recommended amount of fish oils, Sally is able to choose the right amounts and types of fish to eat, using a list similar to the one in the next section. (1 gram = 0.035 oz. To convert grams into ounces, divide by 28.3. For example, 2.4 grams = 0.084 ounces, and 3.6 grams = 0.126 ounces.)

The best source of w-3 fatty acids is fish, and cold-water fish are the best. These include sardines, mackerel and herring. All fish has fish oils in varying amounts. Use the following table to work out your daily or weekly consumption of fish oils. Then compare your daily fish oil consumption with the amount you need to consume for good health.

The content of fish oils in fish

	W-3 fish oils per 100 g raw fish
Atlantic salmon, mackerel	2.0, 2.5 g (2000–2500 mg)
Herring, tuna, rainbow trout, sardines (canned in oil, drained)	1.0–1.7 g (1000–1700 mg)
Ocean perch, snapper, whiting, striped mullet	approx. 0.3 g (300 mg)

Source: USDA Nutrient Database for Standard Reference

Work out your daily fish oil requirement

Step 1: Your average daily energy requirements (see page 45) = _____ kilojoules.

Step 2: Multiply your daily energy requirements by 0.3 and again by 0.04 = _____ = fish oil kilojoules.

Step 3: Fish oil kilojoules _____ divided by 37 = _____ = daily fish oil needs in grams.

To convert grams to ounces, divide by 28.3.

Compile a list of some fish meal ideas, with the aim of increasing the amount of fish oils in your diet. Here are a couple of suggestions to start you off:

FISH	MEAL IDEA
Tuna	Tuna salad
Salmon	Grilled with fresh dill

Incorporate these and other fish meals in your diet. Aim for at least three fish meals a week.

General guidelines for obtaining more essential fatty acids

To increase your intake of w-3 fatty acids, eat more:

✓   Fish, in particular cold-water fish.
✓   Green leafy vegetables.
✓   Flax seeds, linseed oil, soybean oil, walnut oil, canola oil.
✓   Brazil nuts, walnuts: six to ten daily.
✓   Seed sprouts.

To increase your intake of w-6 fatty acids, eat more:

✓   Green leafy vegetables.
✓   Corn, safflower, sunflower, walnut, sesame and soybean oils.
✓   Seed sprouts.
✓   Seeds and nuts

Practical hints for taking in essential fatty acids

✓   Cook with canola, soy or walnut oils.
✓   Add walnuts to salads.
✓   Use cold-pressed flaxseed oil in salads.
✓   Don't heat oils to smoking temperature if frying.

Antioxidants

To find out if your diet is adequate in essential fatty acids, visit:
www.nutrition4health.com.au

A diet rich in antioxidants reduces the chances of heart disease. They are beneficial to our health, as they prevent harmful chemical reactions from occurring. Antioxidants are abundant in fruit and vegetables, tea, wine and legumes.

✅ Include 400–500 grams, or about a pound of fruit and vegetables in your diet each day. That's two to three serves each
of fruit and vegetables. Aim for maximum variety.

✅ Include legumes such as lentils and dried beans in your diet.

You'll find more information on antioxidants in Chapter 6.

Wine: the French paradox

Scientists looking at heart disease patterns around the world noticed that
the French population had much lower rates of heart disease compared
with the rest of the world. Yet the French had similar risk factors and
cholesterol levels to people living in the UK. Studies that examined the
differences between the diets of the French and the English found that the
higher consumption of wine by the French stood out as the most plausible
explanation. More studies were then undertaken to try and explain this
'French Paradox'.

It became clear that the alcohol content of wine per se wasn't the
answer, as beer and spirits failed to produce the same results. It appeared
that wine held the answer. Extracts of red wine were analysed in an
attempt to find the answer. Two interesting groups of bioactive molecules
were found: anthocyanins and polyphenols. Anthocyanins were traced
back to the seeds of the grape, and the polyphenols were derived from
the skins. These two groups of chemicals were shown to have beneficial
effects on blood chemistry. These effects can be summarised as follows:

✅ They have strong antioxidant properties, and prevent the formation
of free radicals.

✅ They prevent clumping of platelets (the cells responsible for forming
blood clots).

✅ They help to keep blood circulating smoothly in the arteries.

✅ They reduce the damage caused by LDL cholesterol.

How much wine is optimal?

The following amounts showed the most benefit:

- For women, up to two standard drinks per day.
- For men, up to three standard drinks per day.

One standard drink is 100 millilitres (3 ½ fl oz) of wine.

Drinking more than the optimal amount doesn't provide any further benefit; in fact, the reverse is true. Drinking more than two standard drinks a day for women, and more than four standard drinks a day for men, increases the risk of heart disease. It is possible to have too much of a good thing!

Red vs white

Red wine is a better source of polyphenols, with white wine having a much lower amount. Grape juice has half the amount of polyphenols found in red wine. This still makes it an excellent source of these antioxidants, and of course it has no alcohol.

Coffee

Recent research into coffee and its effects on heart health have resulted in a mixed bag of findings. However, some facts are available. The key players are diterpenes (cafestol and kahwed) which are naturally present in the coffee bean. Cafestol and kahwed have the ability to increase cholesterol levels.

These substances find their way out of the coffee bean and into the cup of coffee with the help of boiling water. They are retained by a coffee filter. Therefore, instant granulated coffee and filtered coffee don't contain cafestol or kahwed and don't raise cholesterol levels. Scandinavian, Italian, Turkish and Greek coffee, on the other hand, were shown to raise cholesterol levels.

Diterpenes raise total cholesterol, LDL cholesterol and triglycerides, and lower HDL cholesterol.

Not everyone who drinks coffee has a high cholesterol level, but if your cholesterol level is high I encourage you to limit your intake of Scandinavian, Italian, Turkish or Greek coffee. The increase in cholesterol is significant—coffee could be responsible for your cholesterol reading 6.5 mmol, which is 1 mmol above the recommended upper figure of 5.5 mmol.

Caffeine doesn't raise cholesterol. If you are looking for a caffeine boost, drink instant or filtered coffee, and reserve your favourite cup of coffee for a time when you can truly enjoy it. Overall, aim not to drink more than five cups of coffee a day.

chapter six

Tuning your immune system

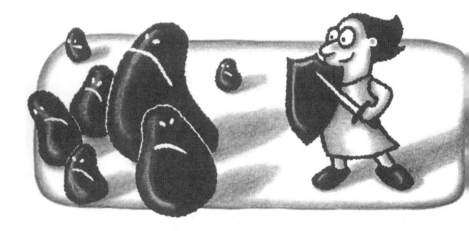

GOAL

- To optimise your immune system by maintaining an adequate level of nutrients in your diet

BENEFITS

- You will spend less time 'soldiering on' in pain and discomfort due to chronic infections

- You'll be less likely to catch colds, flu and other bugs from others

- You will enjoy more pain-free days

The role of nutrition in immunity

The immune system is a complex array of chemical warfare. In order to maintain health, our body relies on a defence system that is swift-acting and accurate in reaching its target. Every day, our immune system faces bacteria, viruses, fungi and other invading bugs. Whether or not these develop into an infection that has you bedridden or sniffling around the office is very much dependent on how well you look after your immune system. The beneficial role of nutrition in immunity is only recently being recognised. Scientists are beginning to look to nutrition as antibiotics fail to kill new resistant strains of bacteria, and viruses mutate faster than we can produce vaccines. Many scientists are faced with the realisation that it may come down to the immune system alone to fight its battles. Nutrition will often make a difference as to whether or not your immune system will fight infections or succumb to them.

Although our food supply is plentiful, there is an oversupply of highly refined, nutritionally compromised foods. Food processing has mass-produced numerous food items loaded with energy, but with little nutritional value. This has made it possible for us to feed our hunger and satisfy our cravings, yet leave our body malnourished. Imbalances and deficiencies of nutrients may result in harmful effects on the body's immune system, which can manifest in frequent colds, flu or chronic fatigue. Some of the effects of poor nutrition on the immune system are:

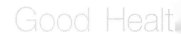
- Fewer white cells (fighter cells) available to fight invading bugs.
- Fewer antibodies (defence artillery) against bacteria and viruses.
- Poorer communication between the fighter cells and antibodies due to decreased messenger chemicals—this may be compared to a trained fighter pilot being given a horse to ride into battle.

An adequate diet rich in nutrients that boost the immune function can prevent these deleterious effects on the immune system. We will now look at the nutrients necessary for a robust immune system.

Antioxidant defences

In order to grow, repair and move, the human body needs energy. We have evolved a system of harnessing energy which is essentially one of combusting or burning 'food'. This process is vital for our very survival; however, it does have side effects. It produces free radicals, unstable molecules that carry tiny electrical charges and attract other molecules—an analogy is a static comb attracting hair. Free radicals are capable of changing chemical structures. For most bodily structures, even a small change in its chemistry means a change in its function. Free radical damage may occur to tissues such as elastin, or skin protein structures, enzymes, hormones, lipids, proteins, unsaturated fatty acids and DNA (our genetic blueprint). In addition to those generated by body metabolism, free radicals can also be ingested or inhaled as environmental pollutants (such as by smoking), or are generated during the metabolism of some types of drugs. So, in an increasingly more polluted environment, our bodies are exposed to a larger battery of free radicals.

Circumstances which increase the need for antioxidant intake

It's particularly important to include a good dose of antioxidants in your daily diet if you identify with any of the following:

- Smoking*
- Stress**
- Increased exposure to car fumes
- Poor dietary habits, especially poor vegetable and fruit intake
- Excessive exposure to UV rays
- Alcohol

Hereditary conditions:

- Family history of heart disease
- Diabetes
- Genetically excessive iron absorption

* You need extra vitamin C-rich fruits and vegetables.
** You need to increase the amount of vitamin E in your diet.
(Refer back to Chapter 1 for sources of both vitamins.)

Antioxidants offer protection against:

- Changes in white cell (fighter cell) chemistry.
- Chronic generation of free radicals leading to chronic inflammatory conditions such as arthritis.
- Depressed immune system due to inhalant radicals (as found in cigarette smoke).

Fortunately, there is something we can do to help keep free radicals under tight control. We can provide our body with a healthy supply of antioxidants. Antioxidants come from our diet. How much you need to eat depends on its quality. You may supply your body with enough ammunition against free radicals, or you may just leave yourself short.

In the rest of this section we'll look at some of the key antioxidants and their food sources.

Supplementation isn't the answer

It's essential to note that antioxidants need to interact with each other to cope with free radicals. By joining forces they provide a much stronger defence system against the damage caused by free radicals. Supplementation with any one antioxidant is of limited value compared to the consumption of foods rich in many antioxidants. Some supplements will offer a limited number of antioxidants together—for example, A, C and E vitamins—in order to boost the antioxidant effect. While this is a good idea, keep in mind that the different types of antioxidants are still being identified and most are not available as vitamin pills.

The complete spectrum of antioxidants can only be obtained from a well-balanced diet.

Free radical quenchers

Vitamins C and E, as well as the pro-vitamin β-carotene, are essential to healthy immunity. A deficiency of these vitamins significantly cripples the immune system. Numerous studies show that a deficiency produces a poorer response to antigens. Antigens are proteins present on invading bugs such as bacteria. They are what our immune system is on the lookout for, just like a radar tracking enemy craft. A lack of these three antioxidants causes malfunctions in this detection system. Antigen recognition and destruction is a key feature of our immune system, preventing infections from taking hold and spreading further.

The link between nutrition and viral infections

A study looking at the role of selenium and vitamin E in immune function showed that a deficiency of either one of these allowed a usually dormant virus to turn into an infective type. These findings have scientists thinking that certain nutrient deficiencies allow viruses to become infectious.

Trace elements

Five trace elements form part of the enzymes (molecules that speed up chemical reactions) that are essential for the swift and accurate response of the immune system. Thus, a deficiency of any of these five nutrients will lower our ability to fight infections. The five trace elements are:

- selenium
- iron
- copper
- manganese
- zinc

Is your intake of these five trace elements adequate? Refer to the relevant section in Chapter 1.

Compounds with antioxidant properties

Scientists are just beginning to scratch the surface of the vast collection of antioxidants in foods. The list of known antioxidants is growing, as more accurate and sensitive methods are

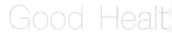
found for deciphering their chemistry. Some well-known groups of antioxidants are:

- Sulphur-containing organic compounds found in garlic and onions.
- Indole alkaloids (indoles, limonoids) and vitamin P (bioflavonoids) found in citrus fruits.
- Monotrenes found in carrots.

Many more are being identified. This is why it would be a mistake to think that you can get antioxidants from a bottle purchased at your health food store. What has been bottled in a laboratory is only a fraction of the full battery of molecules with potent antioxidant properties. Food, (and some food groups in particular), is by far the richest source of antioxidants. Take some time now to look at Checkpoint 8 and check the level of antioxidants in your diet.

checkpoint 8   *Check the level of antioxidants in your diet*

Circle the appropriate answers to the following questions. When you have finished, check the answers below.

How often = how many pieces of fruit or how many serves of vegetables.

	< 1/day	1/day	2/day	>2/day
1. How often do you eat fresh fruit?	a	b	c	d
2. How often do you eat citrus fruit?	a	b	c	d
3. How often do you eat strawberries, mangoes or kiwifruit?	a	b	c	d
4. How often do you drink fresh fruit juice?	a	b	c	d
5. How often do you eat vegetables?	a	b	c	d

	< 1/day	1/day	2/day	>2/day
6. How often do you eat red peppers, tomato or broccoli?˙	a	b	c	d
7. How often do you eat carrots, spinach or sweet potato?	a	b	c	d
8. How often do you eat pumpkin or yellow squash?	a	b	c	d
9. How often do you eat rockmelon, apricots or peaches?	a	b	c	d
10. How often do you use wheatgerm or sunflower oils, or eat nuts or seeds?	a	b	c	d
11. How often do you use soy, corn or a groundnut oil?	a	b	c	d
12. How often do you eat avocado?	a	b	c	d

˙For example, if you eat mangoes three times a week and strawberries four times a week, but you don't eat kiwifruit, then your answer is 'b' (1/day).

ANSWERS

- If you answered 'a' or mostly 'a' to questions 1–4, your diet appears to be low in natural sources of vitamin C.
- If you answered 'a' or mostly 'a' to questions 5–9, your diet appears to be low in natural sources of β-carotene.
- If you answered 'a' or mostly 'a' to questions 10–12, your diet appears to be low in natural sources of vitamin E.

Solutions to the antioxidant shortage

It's easy to have a good amount of antioxidants in your diet, but you may be wondering, 'Where do I start? Which foods are better than others? And what is the best selection?' Follow the guidelines in the next section and I guarantee you will become an expert at selecting the right foods to meet your antioxidant needs. The three musketeers are:

✔ carrots
✔ wheatgerm
✔ citrus fruits

These three foods have very high contents of β-carotene, vitamin E and vitamin C, respectively, together with other antioxidants. Include the three in your diet every day, or use the following substitutions.

Substitutes for carrots

Spinach	Pumpkin	Rockmelon
Sweet potatoes	Tomato	Apricots
Broccoli	Mangoes	Peaches

Substitutes for wheatgerm

Sunflower oil	Avocados	Peanuts	Corn oil
Groundnut oil	Almonds	Pumpkin seeds	Sunflower seeds

Substitutes for citrus fruits

Mangoes	Kiwifruit	Blackcurrants	Strawberries
Tomatoes	Broccoli	Brussel sprouts	Red peppers

LET'S VISIT THE GREENGROCER

The greengrocer or fruit and vegetable markets are the best places to stock up on your antioxidant foods. Look for red, blue-purple and yellow-coloured vegetables and fruit, and green herbs. Check that they are fresh and well stored. Look out for:

- Parsley and thyme (for flavones).
- Onions, kale, broccoli, apples, cherries and berries (for flavonols).
- Citrus fruit (for flavanones).
- Apples, apricots and cherries (for catechins).
- Cherries and grapes (for anthocyanidins).
- Legumes and soy (exclusively for isoflavones).

Rosemary

Spices and herbs are great sources of antioxidants, with rosemary being one of the best. Analysis of rosemary sprigs reveals they contain carnosol, carnosic acid, rosmanol, rosmarinic acid, rosmaridiphenol and rosmariquinone. Carnosic acid is the most powerful antioxidant known, kind of like the stealth fighter prized by the American defence forces. Here are some foods that marry well with rosemary: lamb, pork, poultry, fish, carrots, spinach and zucchini.

Practical manoeuvres in the kitchen

To increase your antioxidant intake:

- Use cold-pressed oils in salads.
- Use fresh herbs.
- Eat fresh vegetables.
- Eat fresh fruit.
- Drink or eat soy-derived foods regularly. Choose from tofu (bean curd), soy milk, miso soup and, of course, soy beans.

Free radicals and aging

The free radical theory of aging is fascinating reading. Although this is not the place to introduce an entire new topic, I would like briefly to share a few scientific discoveries on the subject. Sensitive tests have been developed to estimate the damage caused by free radicals on human DNA, our genetic blueprint. The tests show that there are approximately 10 000 'hits' on human DNA each day. DNA repair enzymes, like workers in a damaged nuclear reactor, try to control any damage by repairing the damaged fractions. Not all of the damage can be stopped. Furthermore, the damage accumulates with age. Or, if we place the cart before the donkey, we look and feel older because there is more radical damage. There is nothing we can do about the passage of time, but slowing down the rate of free radical damage is another story—and nutrition is the key.

Foods that promote free radical formation

- ✗ Smoked meats or smoked fish
- ✗ Char-grilled meats and char-grilled protein-rich foods
- ✗ Animal fat

Foods that prevent free radical formation

If you are fond of barbecued meals, then enjoy your char-grilled meats, chicken or poultry with a combination of foods that prevent free radical formation:

    Fresh green salads

Fresh fruits—aim for at least five different types a day (a fruit platter is a great idea)

✓ Wine in moderation

✓ Tea

✓ Wholegrain cereals and bran

Go easy on antioxidant supplements

Taking antioxidants in excess may well add oil to the fire. There is evidence that supplements in excess of the recommended daily intakes are pro-oxidant, which means that they actually increase free radical formation. *Add colour, not pills, to your diet!*

Foods that move things along in the digestive system prevent the harmful chemical reactions which produce free radicals—this is where high-fibre foods like wholegrain cereals fit in. To get more information on high-fibre foods, visit my website: www.nutrition4health.com.au

Speedy antioxidant boosters

Drinks are often the most easily available nutritional vehicles. They save you time in preparation and have you out of the kitchen in no time. Drinking is faster than eating, and the nutrients are absorbed faster.

A busy schedule and a fast-paced lifestyle may prevent you from cooking a gourmet meal; however, whipping up a nutritious drink shouldn't 'eat' into your day. The benefit from each of the following drinks, which are rich in numerous antioxidants, is a nutrient boost targeted to improve your defence system. Drink up!

Summer Shake

Full of flavonols, flavanones and flavour!

1 cup strawberries

½ seedless orange, peeled well

½ teaspoon honey or maple syrup

❖ Wash strawberries well.

❖ Blend orange with strawberries and honey.

❖ Serve in your favourite glass.

❖ You may wish to strain the juice, but this will lower its nutritional value.

Afternoon Pick-me-up

Full of anthocyanidins

1 cup seedless grapes

½ seedless orange, peeled

❖ Blend or juice both and top with crushed ice.

Instant Reward

A boost of antioxidants

1 large apple, peeled

½ small lemon, peeled

½ cup strawberries

❖ Juice all three in any order.

❖ Serve with crushed ice.

Orange Blaze
More flavanones and flavour!

1 large seedless orange
½ cup peeled, just-ripe pawpaw

❖ Juice or blend the two fruits together.
❖ Serve in your favourite glass with crushed ice.

Kaleidoscope
An antioxidant cocktail

½ cup strawberries
½ cup seedless grapes
½ seedless orange

❖ Blend all fruits well.
❖ Serve in your favourite glass topped with crushed ice.

Try your own combinations, keeping in mind the following antioxidant properties of selected fruit.

For more recipes rich in antioxidants, visit:
www.nutrition4health.com.au

Antioxidant group	Found in
Flavonols	Apples, cherries, berries, tea
Flavanones	Citrus fruit
Catechins	Apples, cherries, tea
Anthocyanidins	Grapes, cherries

chapter seven

Stress and nutrition

■ GOALS

- To avoid a high-fat diet
- To ensure adequate levels of vitamins B and C in your diet
- To limit foods/drinks that induce stress-like effects
- To avoid unsound diets that compromise your health

■ BENEFITS

- You will be more resistant to the effects of chronic stress
- You will be better able to handle stress

Are your eating habits stress-inducing?

Tick the boxes that apply to you.

On average:

☐ I drink more than five cups of coffee daily.

☐ I drink more than four standard drinks a day [for men]

☐ I drink more than two standard drinks a day [for women]

☐ I snack mostly on sweets (e.g. chocolate, pastries, chocolate biscuits)

Also:

☐ I occasionally go on a fast.

☐ I occasionally skip meals.

☐ I follow a macrobiotic diet (comprising only vegetables, fruit and grains).

☐ I follow a diet of less than 6300 kilojoules a day (1500 calories) [for men].

☐ I follow a diet of less than 5040 kilojoules a day (1200 calories) [for women].

If you ticked any of the above boxes, you need to do some repair work on your eating and drinking habits. Each of the above dietary behaviours places stress on your body. Read on to find out why, and what you can do to reduce the harmful effects of these habits.

Diet and stress

The scientific community is divided on the subject of psychological stress and its effects on our physiology, and more importantly on how it affects our nutrient needs. There are those who say that stress doesn't increase our requirements for nutrients, and others who say that it brings about changes to the body's chemistry which lead to higher usage of nutrients, and therefore increases our requirement for them. More and more evidence is accumulating to convince the sceptics that psychological stress— for example, losing a job, or being in a very difficult job—leads to chemical adaptations in the body. A recent study at the Department of Psychology in the University of Antwerp, Belgium, showed that even mild psychological stress (such as sitting for an exam) leads to changes in blood chemistry. Simulation exercises used to train astronauts in Russia (for example, a mock elevation to a height of 8000 metres or 8749 yards) resulted in measurable changes in brain chemicals. Studies looking at the physiological effects of intense periods of stress in the workplace associated with meeting deadlines showed an increase in heart rate and blood pressure, and several similar studies showed that stressed men had relatively higher cholesterol levels. It's not clear if the rise in blood cholesterol is a direct effect of stress or a consequence of eating a higher-fat diet during periods of stress. It may be that both are responsible.

It's clear that some things we consume mimic the effects of stress on our bodies. Severe restrictions on kilojoules and protein may not only compromise our ability to handle stress, but can actually add a significant amount of emotional stress to our life. As evidence continues to accumulate, scientists are becoming more convinced that our eating habits make a significant difference to how we feel and how we cope with stress.

There is no doubt in my mind that nutrition affects how well we cope with stress, and that inadequate nutrition makes it harder to cope both mentally and physically with stress.

Later in this chapter we will consider some dietary guidelines that may be useful in times of stress, but first let's examine some background facts.

Fundamentals of survival: the fight or flight response

In prehistoric times, a caveman had no problem in recognising danger when he saw it: anything bigger than him (a mammoth, say) was rightly perceived as a threat, and his body was instantly ready either to fight or flee from the threat (this is known as the fight or flight response), as the situation required. In scientific terms, the caveman's physiological adaptation was as shown in the following figure.

The flight or fight response

Mammoth ⇨ Adrenalin (stress hormone) ⇨ Increased:
> Heart rate
> Blood pressure
> Breathing
> Blood sugar levels
> Free fatty acids

Whether or not the caveman fought the mammoth and survived, or ran away from it, the outcome was a return to regular breathing, a slower heart rate, and so on. In other words, he could sit in his cave and have a snooze until it was time to hunt the beast for food again.

Nowadays, things are a little less clear—or they *can* be for people involved in psychologically demanding situations day in and day out. Longer working hours, stronger competition and, most of all, very demanding jobs create a background of high emotional stress. To put it simply, there is just no time to have a relaxing snooze after a stressful event. This gradually takes its toll on our physiology, to the point where many people today complain of feeling 'burnt out', 'stressed out', chronically fatigued, and so on. Let's take a closer look at the responses to stress by tracing the pathway of the hormones released in response to stress.

Hormones released in response to stress

1. Stress Adrenalin
2. Stress

           Corticotrophin releasing hormone

                   Adrenocorticotrophic hormone (ACTH)

                  Cortisol

Adrenalin and cortisol are hormones released in response to stress. They increase the number of immune cells (fighter cells) in the blood, which increases the chances of tiny clots forming in the bloodstream, making for a more sluggish circulation as well as increasing our blood sugar levels, heart rate, breathing rate and blood pressure.

All of these adaptations are designed to make it easier for us either to escape or fight. In other words, our response to stress is the same as the caveman's, yet the sources of the stress are often different. It's important to recognise, however, that stress in the form of emotional stress—for example, a tense situation at work or at home—will lead to a set of responses that are very similar to those produced by physical stress. The main difference between the two types of stress responses is the time frame. Instead of evoking an immediate response to physical danger, mental stress keeps us in a state of less dramatic but prolonged tension. The release of cortisol into the bloodstream usually down-regulates the body's hormones, or brings them back to normal to end the tension; however, chronic stress can throw this hormonal control out of whack. The body develops a state of hyperactivity where the timely return to a calmer state is missing. The physical effects of long-term stress on our body are described by the term 'allostatic load'. The allostatic load, or the results of prolonged stress, include:

- Higher lipid (blood fats) levels.*
- Higher blood sugar levels.
- Higher blood pressure.*
- Increased heart rate.

* Risk factors for heart disease.

Dietary means to counteract the effects of chronic stress

Diet can help to limit the physiological effects of chronic stress, namely increased blood levels of fat and sugar, and to provide sufficient amounts of the B-complex vitamins.

EAT A DIET LOW IN FAT—IN PARTICULAR, LOW IN SATURATED FAT

Eating a diet low in fat will prevent high blood fat levels. Go back to Chapter 4 and have another look at Checkpoint 4, where you calculated how much fat you eat, then refer to the appendix for some suggestions regarding nutritious low-fat meals to choose when dining out.

EAT REGULAR MEALS TO REGULATE YOUR BLOOD SUGAR LEVELS

Try to get into a routine of eating regular meals. For between-meal snacks, eat a piece of fruit or any of the snacks in the left-hand column of the list below.

AVOID DRINKING SWEET BEVERAGES AND EATING SWEETS

There is too much sugar in beverages like soft drinks and fruit drinks. Unless you go for a long walk or a run after consuming foods that are high in sugar, the excess amount of sugar will elevate your blood sugar levels, call on a hormone called insulin, and promote fat gain. Use the following guide to keep your sugar intake optimal.

Satisfying a sweet tooth in a nutritious way

Choose	Avoid
Fresh fruit, fruit canned in unsweetened juice	Lollies, chocolate, toffees
Plain biscuits	Chocolate-coated biscuits, cream cakes, pastries, fruit pies
Raisin or fruit bread, light fruit muffins, scones with jam	Doughnuts, tortes, cheesecake
Fat-reduced yoghurt, or fruit sorbets, lite ice-cream, lite soy desserts	Regular ice-cream, rich ice-cream
Low-fat frais fromage	Mousse, cream-based desserts

ENSURE ADEQUATE LEVELS OF VITAMINS B_6 AND B_1

Vitamin B_6 is part of an enzyme that helps to make serotonin, the neurotransmitter that brings about a sensation of calm and makes us feel relaxed. Research shows that a lack of vitamin B_6 leads to overall heightened psychological distress or, in simple terms, makes us feel on edge. Long-term deficiency of this vitamin can result in depression, fatigue and confusion.

Vitamin B_1 is also essential for a composed and energetic mood. In one study, people supplemented with vitamin B_1 performed tasks faster and were generally more clear-headed. This may be related to the vitamin's crucial role in helping to transmit nerve impulses. Refer back to Chapter 1 for the best sources of these two vitamins.

Dietary components that imitate stress reactions

Some dietary constituents consumed in excess may increase the allostatic load—that is, the physiological effects of chronic stress. These include caffeine and alcohol.

CAFFEINE

The body responds to caffeine by releasing adrenalin, which, as you may recall, increases blood sugar levels and circulating blood fats, quickens the heart rate and elevates blood pressure.

In our caveman/mammoth example of the effects of stress, we could substitute caffeine for the mammoth and end up with a similar scenario. It's difficult to think of a cappuccino or latté as a source of stress; however, the cascade of chemical reactions is very similar, and the body has no way of recognising the difference. If you drink coffee, your body will produce adrenalin (a stress hormone) in response. The body's chemistry changes in the same way, regardless of whether the increase in adrenalin is a result of a stressful situation at the office or a cup of your favourite coffee.

Recent research indicates that drinking in excess of five cups of drip coffee a day, which equates with consuming over

687 milligrams of caffeine, is associated with an increased like-lihood of a heart attack.

A milder side effect of drinking coffee in excess is dehy-dration. Drinking five cups of coffee has been shown to result in fluid losses of up to 1.3 litres (2.3 pints [UK], 2.7 pints [US]), representing mild dehydration. This is enough to give some people a symptomatic headache or to bring on fatigue, making it more difficult for them to cope with their daily tasks. It's a good idea to drink a glass of water for every cup of coffee you drink, to replace the extra body fluid you will lose.

> Consume a glass of water for every cup of coffee you drink.

ALCOHOL

Drinking alcohol increases blood pressure, heart rate, breathing and blood fats. Again, these are the classic physiological responses to perceived stress. Like caffeine, alcohol has the potential to place undue stress on the body. The scientific and popular lit-erature sometimes refers to the metabolism of alcohol as 'detoxification', using phrases like 'the liver detoxifies the alco-hol in the blood'. Clearly, this implies a poisonous substance. Some long-term signs of drinking too much alcohol are inflam-mation of the stomach, frequent infections and liver damage. Consuming alcohol in excess places heavy demands on your body, and chronic excessive drinking is a serious threat to both physiological and psychological well-being.

Although alcohol is potentially harmful, for most healthy people drinking alcohol *in moderation* will do no harm, and there is some solid evidence that drinking wine has a beneficial effect on our heart health (see Chapter 5). For most people, alcohol consumption has been shown to have no ill-effects on health if limited to a maximum of four standard drinks a day for men and two standard drinks a day for women. A standard drink contains about 10 grams (⅓ oz) of pure alcohol. Examples of standard drinks are:

- A pint of light beer (425 millilitres or approximately 15 fl oz).
- A schooner of regular beer (285 millilitres or approximately 10 fl oz).
- A schooner of wine cooler (285 millilitres or approximately 10 fl oz).
- A small glass of wine (120 millilitres or approximately 4⅕ fl oz).
- A port or sherry (60 millilitres or approximately 2 fl oz).
- A nip of spirits or liqueurs (30 millilitres or approximately 1 fl oz).

The pick-me-up nutrients

Let's face it: most people overdo it at one time or another. The queazy feeling in the stomach, the unbearable headache and the parched mouth after a heavy night are signs that we have temporarily over-toxicated our body with alcohol.

On a nutritional level, excessive alcohol intake depletes the body of the following nutrients: potassium, magnesium, vitamin C, the B vitamins, zinc and calcium. Replenishing these is therefore a priority. Even if you have no appetite, you should still be able to drink, so sip on fruit or vegetable juice. By drinking fruit or vegetable juices, you are replenishing your body's vitamin C, potassium, magnesium and some of the B vitamins. The zinc and calcium will have to wait until your body is ready for something more solid. I recommend that you have something light to eat that is rich in the nutrients you have depleted your body of. Avoid eating fatty foods. Fats are much harder to digest and cause food to sit in the stomach longer—something your stomach doesn't want if you have a hangover. Suggestions to help as a pick-me-up are:

✓ Bread and yeast extract spreads, which are excellent sources of vitamin B, potassium and magnesium.

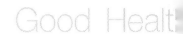

✓ Vegetables, which are an excellent source of vitamins B and C, magnesium and potassium—a salad is an excellent choice.
✓ Grilled fish and salad.

Rigid dieting

While reducing your body weight is beneficial to your health if you are overweight, how you go about it is crucial to your well-being. Diets that overly restrict your energy intake lead to increased anxiety. In the long term, unbalanced dieting behaviour is harmful and may result in disordered eating. A recent study looking at the effects of dieting in women linked very low kilojoule diets to the reduced production of serotonin—the 'happy' brain neurotransmitter—due to a shortage of tryptophan in the diet. A chronic under-supply of tryptophan may result in depression.

Stressful effects of unwise dieting

- Limited food choices can lead to anxiety about eating in social situations, and to food cravings for people following a diet of less than 5040 kilojoules (1200 calories) for women and less than 6300 kilojoules (1500 calories) for most men.
- Skipping meals to hasten weight loss leads to fatigue and irritability.

Discussing your weight goals with a qualified nutritionist to work out a weight-management program will help you to reach your goal weight faster without compromising your health and lifestyle.

The fable of the hare and the tortoise applies well to weight reduction. A successful weight-reduction program allows for:

- Social occasions which include your favourite foods.
- Sufficient intake of kilojoules to prevent a slowing down of the metabolic rate.
- A balanced intake of nutrients in order to prevent nutrient deficiencies.
- A steady reduction in weight that is noticeable within a few weeks in terms of how your clothes fit.

While weight reduction requires motivation, it doesn't have to be stressful!

> You will find useful guidelines and individual feedback if you are attempting to lose weight by visiting my website:
> www.nutrition4health.com.au

chapter eight

Nutrition and brain performance

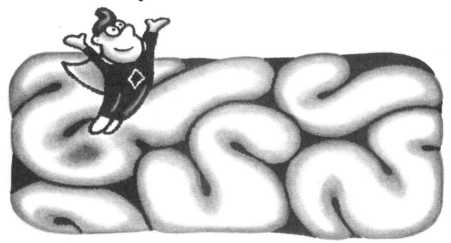

■ GOALS

- To keep your blood sugar levels steady throughout the day

- To know which foods will prevent sluggishness and/or sleepiness

- To know which foods will help you to wind down and sleep better

- To optimise your intake of B group vitamins and choline

■ BENEFITS

- You will optimise your memory recall and decision-making

- You will stay alert longer

- You will avoid periods of vagueness, feeling drowsy and sleepy following lunch

- You will avoid periods of poor concentration

- You will wind down faster and sleep better

Food and brain chemistry

Improving your nutrition offers a means of improving cognitive function. If you suffer from poor eating habits, changes to your diet can improve your ability to concentrate, recall events and make quick decisions. The composition of your meals may help you to wind down and 'recharge your batteries' faster. Improving your brain performance doesn't require an exotic diet and supplemental potions. The dietary changes that are beneficial to brain performance are easy to make and, what's more, fall within the balanced guidelines for overall health. They are based on an understanding of how nutrition influences the brain, and on the recognition that brain chemistry may influence brain performance.

The brain is a tight network of neurons, or nerve cells. Our cognition—our recognition of what's happening inside and around us—is based on the communication between millions of these brain cells. The communication is made possible by tiny electrical currents. An electrical current passing along the nerve cell causes it to fire and release tiny messenger molecules called neurotransmitters. These messenger chemicals released by one nerve cell jump on to the next nerve cell and then the next, each time causing another nerve cell to fire off. The junction between the nerve cells is called a synapse. Scientists are now able to look at the activities in a synapse in many areas of the brain, and this type of research is bringing us close to an understanding of how the brain works and what it needs to function well.

Scientists now know that some neurotransmitters can be recycled with minimum wastage, while others must be made from scratch. Nutrition plays a leading part in the ongoing manufacture of three major neurotransmitters: acetylcholine, adrenalin and serotonin. All three are made in the brain from raw materials supplied by certain foods.

There is an active process of selection between the blood and the brain across a specialised layer of cells called the blood/brain barrier. The blood/brain barrier provides protection against toxic molecules, while helping with the entry of molecules essential for the brain's activity. The mix of nutrients in the bloodstream has a lot to do with what nutrients enter the brain and in what amounts. This, in turn, depends on the food we consume. Here is a quick summary of the effects on the brain of carbohydrates, fats, proteins (amino acids) and alcohol.

CARBOHYDRATES
The brain burns fuel like a V8 engine. About two-thirds of the glucose—the preferred body fuel—available to the entire body will be sequestered by the brain from the bloodstream after a meal. This is because the brain relies on glucose almost exclusively for all the processing it needs to do, and there is a lot to do. It has no way of storing glucose and relies solely on the glucose available in the bloodstream. Adequate blood sugar levels are therefore crucial for optimum cognitive function.

FATS
Fats, or fatty acids, are the structural components of the brain. They are the bricks and mortar for the nerve cells—in particular, for the nerve cells' membranes. Essential fatty acids are needed for healthy brain development. In addition, some are raw materials for neurotransmitters or brain messengers.

AMINO ACIDS
Amino acids, which are the components of proteins, are also required for neurotransmitter synthesis. Tryptophan is an essential amino acid which is turned into the neurotransmitter serotonin

in the brain. Tyrosine, another essential amino acid, is the raw material for dopamine and norepinephrine neurotransmitters (more on this later). In addition, approximately 10 per cent of amino acids are metabolised into glucose for energy.

ALCOHOL

In general, the effect of alcohol on the cognitive function is to impair coordination, perception and sustained attention. Alcohol has no known benefits in terms of the brain's performance, and a well-known and deserved reputation for destroying brain cells.

Meal composition

Research carried out over the last two decades shows that the composition of our meals can influence our mood. This research is ongoing; however, the findings to date may be summarised as follows:

- A meal *high in carbohydrate*—that is, mostly made up of pasta, rice, breads or other starches—increases the uptake of tryptophan, and therefore the amount of serotonin, into the brain. This has been shown to have a calming effect on men and a sleep-inducing effect on women.
- A meal *high in protein*—that is, mostly made up of meat, poultry, fish, eggs or dairy products—increases the uptake of tyrosine, the amino acid precursor of catecholamines. Catecholamines, in contrast to serotonin, help to keep us alert. This is the meal of choice should you want to be as sharp as possible.
- A meal *high in fat*—for example, deep-fried foods, or foods smothered in creamy sauces—will bring on hyper-satiety

syndrome, a rather fancy term for overeating. Fats require long periods of digestion, and the physiological symptoms are feelings of sluggishness, a semi-sleep-like state which is the body's way of telling us it needs to do some serious digesting and would rather not move, or even think for that matter.

Meal times

THE IMPORTANCE OF BREAKFAST

Skipping breakfast is common these days, and the most common reason is lack of time. Yet a number of well-designed studies have shown that having no food in the morning leads to poorer cognitive performance. Missing breakfast can slow down your reaction times and reduce your immediate word recall and spatial memory. For example, you may find that it takes you longer to complete a memorandum at work, or you may search in vain for the name of someone to whom you have just been introduced. This may lead you to conclude that your memory is like a sieve and you are just getting old.

Skipping breakfast is even more detrimental for children, so if you have a young family you should consider eating breakfast with them to set a good example—children really do learn from watching you, and they will pick up your bad habits just as easily as your good ones.

Skipping breakfast
slows down problem-
solving ability.

Good, quick choices for breakfast

- Wholemeal cereal with low-fat milk and a few nuts.
- Toast and peanut butter (no need for extra butter or margarine).

- Toast and lean ham with fat-reduced cheese melted (no butter or margarine).
- Toast and baked beans.
- Fruit and yoghurt if you are in a real hurry.

AVOIDING THE POST-LUNCH DIP

'Post-lunch dip' refers to the onset of sleepiness that many people experience within an hour or so of eating lunch. The post-lunch dip is influenced by our circadian rhythm, which is the name for the daily variations in sleep or how sleepy we feel at certain times of the day and night. One way of looking at the biology behind the circadian rhythm is to consider the variations in cortisol during the day, keeping in mind that the more cortisol we have, the more awake we feel. What you will notice from the graph below is that the cortisol level rises sharply in the early hours of the morning and then declines, hitting a low at around midday. This drop in cortisol is responsible for a drop in our energy levels around lunchtime.

People who work under a lot of stress may not notice the post-lunch dip. Stress, as you may recall, increases cortisol production, and therefore overrides the natural cortisol decline

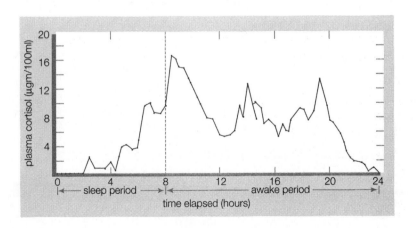

Source: E. D. Weitzman et al., *Journal of Clinical Endocrinology and Metabolism*, vol. 33.

around midday. This is a coping mechanism and a rather short-term measure, because in the long run you are likely to run into chronic fatigue.

As you know, the nutritional composition of a meal will also influence your energy levels. Some meal choices are more likely than others to make you feel like taking a nap, or to sap your energy for quick decision-making.

To avoid a severe post-lunch dip:

✓ Avoid overeating.
✓ Don't skip breakfast, as you are then more likely to overeat at lunch.
✓ Avoid meals that are high in fat.
✓ Avoid sweets or sweetened drinks.
✓ Eat a low- to moderate-fat meal with some carbohydrate and a good serving of lean protein.

Nutritious lunch choices

✓ Exotic sandwiches—go without butter/margarine and instead choose spreads such as cranberry sauce, mustard, mayonnaise, mint jelly or avocado to complement your sandwich. Choose lean fillings such as ham deluxe, shaved chicken, chilli chicken breast fillet, salmon, tuna or roast turkey. Select a colourful mix of fresh salad vegetables.
✓ Wraps, Turkish bread, pita or focaccia with fillings as above.
✓ Sushi.
✓ Any from the meal choices listed in the appendix.

WINDING DOWN IN THE EVENING

A high-carbohydrate meal or snack is ideal in the evening when winding down after a long day's work. For busy parents, choose a meal with lean meat, chicken or fish, generous amounts of vegetables, and moderate amounts of rice, pasta, potato or similar starches. If you are a vegetarian, substitute legumes for the meat proteins. Avoid high-fat sauces or fatty choices for dinner, as they are more likely to make you feel tired or drowsy and it will be harder for you to go through the routine of putting your children to bed. In addition to robbing you of energy, they will add inches to your waistline. Once the kids are in bed, have a nutritious high-carbohydrate snack to help you wind down. Fruit salad with fat-reduced yoghurt or ice-cream is ideal.

KEEP YOUR MEALS REGULAR
Under normal conditions the brain runs exclusively on glucose. The amount of glucose is tightly regulated in the bloodstream and its level depends primarily on your diet, namely:

- The timing of your meals.
- The amount and type of carbohydrate you eat.

The aim is to achieve a steady supply of sugar to the brain, and the best way to do this is to eat regular meals containing complex carbohydrates. Complex carbohydrate foods such as breads, pasta, rice and other grains keep your blood sugar levels stable by releasing a steady supply of sugar as they are digested. This keeps the brain happy; it processes information faster and recalls information better than a brain that is deprived of sugar. People with low blood sugar levels have much slower reaction times on tests used to assess brain function.

AVOID 'HITTING THE WALL'
'Hitting the wall' is an expression used in athletics. It's an apt description of those times when the blood sugar levels take a

dive and the athlete is overcome by a sudden and extreme tired-ness. It usually occurs during endurance events, such as the marathon, when the athlete is unable to rest or refuel. You may not be running marathons, but you can 'hit the wall' and experience extreme *mental* tiredness if you try to do too much brain work without adequate sustenance. Nowadays, athletes follow special nutritional regimes prior to important events, and even during periods of training. This would ideally be low Glycaemic Index choices—we will be looking at the Glyceamic Index of carbohydrate rich foods on page 132. These regimes, which have been shown to improve performance significantly, are designed to provide the muscles with a steady supply of glucose. It's not surprising, then, that the brain, which relies exclusively on sugar as a fuel, is even more sensitive to falls in blood sugar levels.

The following graphs show the effect of mealtimes on blood sugar levels. Don't forget that you need to eat some complex carbohydrate at each meal for optimal effect.

The effects of irregular mealtimes on blood sugar levels

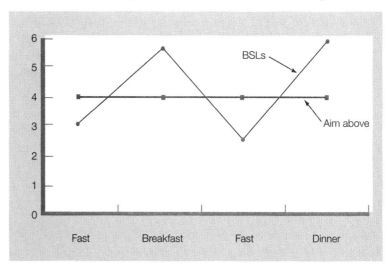

The effects of regular mealtimes on blood sugar levels

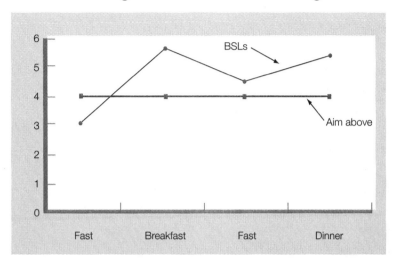

Refuelling station: nutritious complex carbohydrate snacks

If you are in a hurry and can't find the time for a proper meal, these snacks will tie you over until your next meal.

- ✔ Bowl of cereal with low-fat milk.
- ✔ Wholegrain banana jaffle.
- ✔ Raisin toast with a glass of low-fat milk.
- ✔ Fruit smoothie.
- ✔ Cup of vegetable soup with a wholemeal roll.

Some more nutritious snacks

Replace fatty snacks with any from the following list. They are listed from the lowest in fat to the highest in fat.

- fresh fruit
- fruit salad
- fruit kebabs
- fresh vegetables (e.g. ripe tomatoes, carrot sticks)
- dried fruit
- fruit ices
- sorbets
- low-fat yoghurt
- low-fat soft-serve ice-cream
- low-fat ice-cream and fresh fruit
- raisin toast
- cruskets
- rice snacks (97 per cent fat-free) with salsa
- vegetable soup (avoid 'cream of' soups)
- sushi
- yeasty breads and buns with apples or dried fruit
- pancakes with maple syrup
- nuts (approximately ten daily)
- seeds (approximately two tablespoons daily)

Reactive hypoglycaemia

Reactive hypoglycaemia is sometimes described as increased insulin sensitivity. It refers to a higher than normal secretion of insulin following a meal or snack containing carbohydrate. Insulin is a hormone responsible for lowering blood sugar levels, and if over-produced will cause a dangerously low ('hypo') blood sugar level. The symptoms of hypoglycaemia are trembling hands, faintness, confusion and dizziness.

The number of people suffering from this condition is relatively small, although some sources estimate that three out of ten young women have reactive hypoglycaemia. If you do suffer from this condition, avoid eating foods that will cause a rapid rise in blood sugar levels. The glycaemic index of foods is a handy tool to help you achieve this aim.

The glycaemic index of foods

The glycaemic index (GI) offers a way to measure the effect of carbohydrate-rich foods on our blood sugar levels. The glycaemic index ranks foods according to their ability to increase blood sugar levels two to three hours after eating. As you know, sugar and starch both increase the level of glucose—the form that sugar takes in our bloodstream. However, they don't do so at the same speed. For example, pasta produces a much slower rise than potato or rice.

Over 300 foods have now been assigned a GI number, and the list is still growing. A food with a low GI number will cause a slower, steadier rise in glucose levels over a given period of time than similar portions of a food with a higher GI number.

The glycaemic index was originally developed as a tool to help people with diabetes. Diabetes is a condition where glucose levels rise too high and remain elevated for abnormal periods. However, it is also very useful in preventing episodes of reactive hypoglycaemia. Eating low-GI foods will achieve a slow and steady release of glucose into the bloodstream, preventing both the peaks, which cause an abnormally high release of insulin into the bloodstream, and the abnormally low glucose levels which result in uncomfortable symptoms.

HIGH-GI FOODS VERSUS LOW-GI FOODS

Eating meals, and more importantly snacks, with low GI values will help to prevent peaks, followed by sudden dives, in your

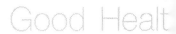

blood sugar levels. Use the following guide to food selection based on their GI values.

A guide to food selection based on GI values

Choose more often	Avoid/eat less often
Untoasted muesli, porridge, Special K, Sultana Bran	Cornflakes, Rice Bubbles, Coco Pops
Mixed grains, fruit loaf, pita bread Wholemeal, wholegrain crispbreads	Bagel, white bread, croissant, crumpet
	Puffed crispbread, rice cakes
Plain biscuits	Plain refined biscuits
Barley, buckwheat, pasta, basmati rice	Regular white rice
	Taco shell
Apple, cherries, peaches, pears, plums	Pineapple, watermelon, rockmelon

Overcoming sleep problems

Our natural sleep pattern is determined primarily by the circadian rhythm, which is in turn governed by light and darkness, or day and night variations. Our sleep pattern is also altered by a number of other factors, including the nutritional components caffeine and amino acids.

CAFFEINE

One well-known effect of coffee is its ability to keep us awake. Studies on the effects of caffeine on sleep have shown that 100 milligrams of caffeine (an average cup of coffee) postpones sleep on average by 15 minutes. This is of course very individual and will depend on whether or not you are a heavy drinker of coffee.

Keep in mind that a cup of coffee contains between 70 and 150 milligrams of caffeine, while carbonated drinks contain around 36 milligrams per 375-millilitre can.

The case for drinking tea

Recent studies looking at the effects of tea drinking have come up with a number of interesting findings. Drinking tea was found to go hand in hand with higher energy levels and reduced anxiety. People performed better within ten minutes of drinking tea, while without a drink of tea their overall alertness declined steadily over the day. Interestingly, drinking coffee didn't have the same effect. Scientists are now looking for what causes these beneficial effects.

AMINO ACIDS

The amino acid composition of a meal may influence our sleeping pattern. The key player here is the amino acid tryptophan. A meal that helps tryptophan to enter the brain will make us feel more drowsy and sleepy and will help us to fall asleep faster. This is because tryptophan is converted into serotonin, the calming-down, 'happy' neurotransmitter. Tryptophan is one of the least available amino acids in the diet. A meal high in protein contains a lot more of the other amino acids, which compete for entry across the brain/blood barrier, essentially bumping off tryptophan. So, eating a meal high in protein will temporarily reduce the chances of tryptophan getting inside the brain, with the end result being less serotonin. Eating a meal high in carbohydrate, on the other hand, helps to carry the tryptophan into the brain. The best sequence of events, therefore, is to have a high-carbohydrate snack sometime after a dinner that includes protein-rich foods.

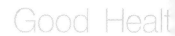

If you are having trouble winding down and falling asleep:

✓ Eat a high-carbohydrate snack for supper—for example, stewed fruit with low-fat ice-cream or custard, fruit and yoghurt, plain wholemeal biscuits, carrot cake or raisin toast.

✓ Try some gentle exercise or a relaxing activity to take your mind off things.

✓ Avoid coffee, strong tea or carbonated beverages later than lunchtime.

Improve your memory with choline

The neurotransmitter acetylcholine is essential for good memory. A number of studies have shown that eating foods rich in choline results in more choline getting inside the brain and more acetylcholine being produced. Just how well this can boost our memory is still unknown, but studies with university students showed that they memorised lists better after taking choline supplements.

Choline is present in a variety of foods, and all natural fats contain some choline. Surveys show that the amount of choline we eat varies between 250 milligrams (0.00875 oz) and 1 gram (0.035 oz) a day. The Food and Nutrition Board (part of the National Academy of Sciences) recently issued recommendations for daily amounts of choline to be supplied in the diet: 550 milligrams (0.01925 oz) daily for men and 425 milligrams (0.014875 oz) daily for women.

If necessary, choline can also be made in the liver from the amino acids methionine and serine with the help of folic acid and vitamin B_{12}. A lack of dietary choline may compromise memory in people who severely limit their fats or are deficient in folic acid and vitamin B_{12}.

If you are considering choline supplementation, bear in mind that it won't offer benefits unless your blood levels of choline are inadequate. It may improve only if you are deficient in choline. Supplements are available in the forms of choline chloride, choline bitartrate and lecithin. Absorption of choline from lecithin is three times more effective than from the other two sources. Be aware that lecithin has some unpleasant side effects if taken in large doses, such as nausea, vomiting and dizziness. Some people develop a 'fishy' smell while taking lecithin. Don't take more than 1 gram ($\frac{1}{30}$ oz) daily. The maximum daily dosage of lecithin before side effects occur is 10 ($\frac{1}{3}$ oz) grams. You may benefit from lecithin supplementation if:

- You drink alcohol in excess of four drinks a day for men, and two drinks a day for women.
- You lack folate and vitamin B_{12} in your diet (refer to the vitamin file in Chapter 1).
- You are following a very low-fat diet.

If you drink alcohol you need more choline, as alcohol destroys choline stores in the liver and possibly in the brain. If you lack folate and vitamin B_{12}, your body is dependent on your diet as the only source of choline. If your diet is low in choline—your diet is extremely low in fat, for example—you don't have a second line of defence.

I recommend a variety of choline-rich foods daily to ensure a good amount of choline in the diet.

Increasing your choline intake

To increase your choline intake, choose:

Wheatgerm	Cauliflower	Green peas	Brewer's yeast
Egg yolk	Lettuce	Soybeans	Lean meats
Spinach	Nuts		

Looking after your nutrition needs

Most people can improve their nutrition through some simple strategies. For some this may mean including more fish in your diet; for others it may mean including more fruit and vegetables. Start with a small aim and put it into practice. It helps if you set weekly or monthly goals. You may, for example, realise that you don't eat enough fish and resolve that in the next week you will eat three fish meals. Having achieved the goal to eat three fish meals for a week, make it a monthly goal and continue until it becomes second nature.

In setting your aims, start with three that would most significantly improve your nutrition. Hopefully you identified some shortcomings in your diet as you read through each of the chapters. Here are some of the most important messages from this book, each of which will help you to improve your nutrition (you can use these to set personal aims):

- Consume a wider variety of foods.
- Keep your saturated fats nice and low.
- Increase the amount of w-3 fatty acids, the type found in fish.
- Look after antioxidants in your diet by eating a variety of fresh vegetables and fruit—the more natural colour in your diet the more antioxidants it will provide you with.
- Eat nuts regularly in small amounts.
- Eat regular meals to achieve a steady supply of glucose (the fuel for our brains).
- Avoid skipping meals and overeating as a consequence.
- Aim to limit your coffee to a maximum of five cups a day; replace the cups of coffee in excess of five with tea.
- Enjoy alcohol in moderation, and choose wine in preference to spirits.

You may find it helpful to keep a record of your meals and drinks to assess your current nutrition, and to set some goals for the future. Keeping your diary for a week or even four days (two weekdays and one weekend) is sufficient. Rate your diet against the food variety models discussed in Chapter 2, as this will help you to see the major shortcomings in your diet. Then look at each of the goals set at the beginning of each chapter. How did you go? If you would like more help with setting realistic goals aimed at improving your nutrition, consult a qualified nutritionist working in your area or visit my website, www.nutrition4health.com.au The website also contains helpful advice on how to put your aims into practice.

Aim to improve your nutrition through a positive approach to healthy eating and avoid harmful dieting regimes lacking in food variety and very low in kilojoules. Respect your health, avoid all extreme restrictions in your diet and try to avoid making 'losing weight' a preoccupation. Instead, work on improving your health—and a slimmer waistline if you wish—through better nutrition combined with regular exercise. Be realistic and acknowledge that it may take you longer to lose weight if you don't start an extreme diet, but a slow, gradual weight loss while you work on improving your nutrition is a weight loss that you can maintain, thus avoiding yo-yo dieting which lowers your metabolism, is harmful for your health (in particular your heart), and more or less sets you up for a lifetime of frustrating dieting. To avoid falling into the trap of unwise dieting, do seek help from a qualified nutritionist who can guide you in beneficial changes to your eating habits.

Improving your health through better nutrition is about making small changes to your eating habits that you are happy with for a lifetime. Trying new foods is part of this change, and this can be fun both when cooking at home and eating out. Cooking nutritious, tasty meals is easy if you use a little creativity and implement moderate change rather than extreme measures. Adding a variety of wonderful spices and herbs to your food works magically, and replaces the need to use fat to add flavour.

The wonderful variety of fresh fruits and vegetables, grains, low-fat dairy products and lean cuts of meats readily available in our supermarkets make it easy to eat in a nutritious way. And finding nutritious meals on the menu when eating out has become a lot easier, too. International restaurants offer a wonderful mix of nutritious meals, low in saturated fats, and we will look at these in the appendix section which follows. Take advantage of this plentiful variety to improve your nutrition, better your health and enjoy a fruitful life to a ripe old age.

Eating out: practice makes perfect

Dining out has become a way of life. When I ask my clients how often they eat out, the usual answer is between two and five times a week, and that's not including business lunches. Eating out saves time. It can be a lot of fun and can increase food variety, with many restaurants serving very nutritious meals. On the other hand, it can be a quick-fill that may be poor in nutritional quality and food variety. It all depends where you eat and the choices you make.

For people determined to keep to a healthy diet, eating out can be frustrating if they don't know which meals to choose. They may restrict their choice to a few 'safe' meals. This reduces food variety in the long run. Others may lose their resolve when faced with the menu choices.

Some of the reasons why we enjoy eating out include:

- great atmosphere
- great food
- great company
- great wine

Two of these reasons are relevant to any food choices we will make. One reason is the choice of wine—a beverage that, in moderation, can be beneficial to our well-being. The remaining reason is the food selection itself. Do the following exercises to work out your priorities when dining.

Exercise 1

Imagine yourself seated at a table at your favourite restaurant. You are enjoying the relaxed atmosphere while waiting for your meal. When the waiter places your meal—your favourite pasta, say—in front of you, you notice that it's overcooked.

Rate your disappointment out of ten: ____/10

Exercise 2

Imagine yourself back at your favourite restaurant. This time the waiter ushers you to a part of the restaurant where some renovations are being carried out. Your meal is delicious, but the atmosphere is sadly lacking.

Rate your disappointment out of ten: ____/10.

Which scenario did you find most disappointing?

Stop dieting

Paying too much attention to food is the number one side effect of being on a diet. The solution is not to call your attempt to improve your nutrition 'dieting', and to shift some of your attention to the other pleasurable aspects of dining out.

Here are some other negative behaviours associated with 'dieting', as opposed to 'improving your nutrition':

- You might worry ahead of time about which meal to choose from the menu.
- You might feel frustrated if you can't find anything suitable on the menu.
- You might feel deprived, and decide to forget your diet for today.
- You find dieting stressful, so you might decide to give it up as not being good for you.

If any of the above describe you, you may need to refocus your approach. Here are some positive steps to take when dining out while modifying your eating habits:

✔ Enjoy the pleasant atmosphere.

✔ Enjoy the pleasant company.

✔ Choose meals from the menu that will provide you with high nutritional content and good taste, without excess fat (see the following section called 'The art of choosing nutritious meals from the menu').

✔ Remember that it's OK to dine on your favourite foods every now and then, without worrying about their nutritional content.

The art of choosing nutritious meals from the menu

This section of the appendix lists meal suggestions and sample menus from a variety of international cuisines, with the aim of optimising your nutrition while dining out. The goals are to:

✔ Keep fat levels within your daily budget.

✔ Increase your intake of antioxidants.

✔ Increase your intake of w-3 fatty acids.

✔ Continue to enjoy dining out!

GENERAL GUIDELINES FOR MENU SELECTION

These terms mean more fat is used

⬆ au gratin (in cheese sauce)	⬆ beurre blanc
⬆ batter-fried	⬆ buttered
⬆ bearnaise	⬆ creamed
⬆ breaded	⬆ crispy

⇑ deep-fried

⇑ double crust

⇑ en croute

⇑ French-fried

⇑ hollandaise

⇑ pan-fried

⇑ pastry

⇑ prime

⇑ rich

⇑ sautéed

⇑ scalloped (escalloped)

⇑ gravy

⇑ thick sauce

These terms mean less fat is used

⇓ baked

⇓ braised

⇓ broiled

⇓ cooked in its own juices

⇓ grilled

⇓ poached

⇓ roasted

⇓ steamed

⇓ stir-fried

Here are some hints regarding meal and drink selection:

- If you're not sure about a dish, ask the waiter what it contains and how it is cooked.
- Specify that your vegetables be prepared without butter or fatty sauces.
- Ask that your salad be served without dressing, or with the dressing on the side so that you can decide how much to use, or ask for just vinegar or lemon juice.
- Say 'no thanks' to gravy or sauce on the meat.
- Ask for grilled, not fried or battered fish, poultry or meat.
- Ask for fresh bread rolls—avoid garlic bread and herb bread.
- Don't be tempted to have seconds. Remind yourself that this isn't the last time you'll be eating out and you can always come back and have the same meal another time.

- Choose fresh fruit for dessert, if possible.
- Eat slowly and enjoy your meal.
- Don't eat food from habit—if the food disappoints you, leave it on the plate.
- Remind yourself to stop eating when you no longer feel hungry.
- If you drink water with your meal, you will taste more flavours in your food.
- Drink wine only in moderation (i.e. up to two standard drinks for women and up to four for men).
- If drinking alcohol, select a mixed drink with one kilojoule-free ingredient (e.g. scotch and water, or diet coke, vermouth and soda, gin and low-kilojoule bitter lemon).

The art of menu selection

Within your fat budget: enjoy	Only on credit: avoid
Soups	
Consommé, gazpacho, minestrone	Cream soups, soups with meat and chicken
	Croutons
Appetisers	
Vegetable plate with salsa	Paté, quiche Lorraine, stuffed appetisers
Steamed vegetables	Cheese, bacon, salami, smoked meats, olives
Green salads with dressing on the side	Mayonnaise-rich salads: potato, macaroni, tuna
Roasted capsicums, eggplant	Caesar salad, Chicken Kiev, antipasto

Within your fat budget: enjoy	Only on credit: avoid
Meat dishes	
Grilled meats, broiled or flame-cooked	Pastry or batter-dipped meats
Broiled, poached, steamed, roasted, baked	Fried, sautéed, au gratin, escalloped, en croute
Cajun, au jus, Provencal, fruit sauce	Creamed, en casserole, with gravy
120–240 grams (4¼–8½ oz) per serve	Above 240 grams (8½ oz) per serve
Vegetables	
Plain steamed, boiled, baked vegetables	Fries, wedges, roasted, creamed vegetables
	Croquettes, bubble and squeak, buttered noodles
Rice and pasta	
Steamed, boiled plain and with low-fat sauces	Buttered noodles, pasta or fried rice
Breads	
Plain, unbuttered rolls, breadsticks, bagels	Buttered, garlic and herb breads, pizza
Sandwiches with mustard or low-fat mayonnaise in place of butter (see the guide to sauces below)	Focaccia with fatty fillings (e.g. salami and cheese)
Focaccia with turkey breast, avocado and salad and low-fat cheese	
Desserts	
Fruit, sorbets, apple strudel, gelato	Cheesecake, French pastries, mousse

What's in the sauce?

Would a sauce by any other name contain the same amount of fat?

Guide to symbols

⇓ Low in fat or low in saturated fat

⇧ High in saturated fat, the more ⇧, the higher the fat content

⇧⇧⇧   Alfredo

⇧⇧⇧   Bearnaise

⇧⇧⇧   Boscaiolla

⇧⇧⇧   Chantilly

⇧⇧⇧   Hollandaise

⇧⇧⇧   Mustard sauce

⇧⇧   Bechamel

⇧⇧   Mornay (cheese sauce)

⇧   Bolognaise

⇧   Bourguignonne

⇧   Espagnole

⇧   Gravy

⇧   Lyonnaise

⇧   Mushroom sauce (⇧⇧ if on bechamel base)

⇧   Veloute

⇓   Apple sauce

⇓   Marinara

⇓   Neapolitan

⇓   Sweet and sour

⇓   Vinaigrette

⇓   White and red wine sauces

Dining out international style

Italian cuisine

Italian food is loved worldwide. Its nutritional content overall is excellent, though some dishes are too high in fat.

Terms meaning more fat

⬆ Antipasto ('before pasta')—olives, salami, prosciutto

⬆ Cannoli—deep-fried pastry shells

⬆ Cannelloni—pasta tubes filled with meat and cheese and topped with sauce

⬆ Eggplant parmesan—fried eggplant

⬆ Fritto—fried

⬆ Crema—creamed

⬆ Parmigiana—breaded (therefore absorbs more fat)

Terms meaning less fat

⬇ Cacciatore—tomato-based sauce

⬇ Cannellini—white kidney beans

⬇ Fresco—fresh

⬇ Fagioli—white beans

⬇ Florentine—spinach

⬇ Gnocchi—potato or flour-based dumpling

⬇ Insalata—fresh garden salad

⬇ Marsala—broth based cooked with wine

⇩ Primavera—spring style (refers to dishes garnished with raw or lightly cooked fresh vegetables with olive oil)

⇩ Polenta—cornmeal mush usually served with sauce (check that it is not served in a fatty sauce)

⇩ Ravioli—ask for meat or spinach filling and served with Neapolitan sauce

⇩ Risotto—rice cooked in broth and sometimes butter

Thin-crust pizza saves on kilojoules. Both thick and deep-pan pizza crusts are higher in energy per serve.

Pizza toppers: the art of choosing pizza

Within your fat budget: enjoy	Only on credit: avoid
Artichoke hearts	Anchovies (OK in moderation)
Beans	Bacon
Bell peppers (capsicum)	Cabanossi
Crabmeat, calamari	Extra cheese
Corn	Olives
Eggplant slices	Pepperoni
Japaleno peppers	Prosciutto
Mushroom slices	Salami
Onion	Sausage or mince
Pineapple	
Prawns and mussels	
Roasted capsicum	

Italian menu

Appetiser/Salad
Bruscetta
(Fresh tomato basil toast)

Soup
Minestrone

Main
Veal Marsala
Fresh Italian salad

Dessert
Lemon gelato

Greek cuisine

Vegetables, seafood, pulses, traditional cheeses and olive oil are the key ingredients of the Greek cuisine, one of the Mediterranean cuisines.

Terms meaning more fat

⬆ Spanakopita and tyropita—vegetables pies
⬆ Saganaki—thick casseri cheese (fried and sometimes flamed in brandy)
⬆ Baklava
⬆ Feta cheese
⬆ Kalamata olives—high in monounsaturated fats, enjoy in moderation
⬆ Anchovies—high in monounsaturated fats, enjoy in moderation

Terms meaning less fat

⬇ Dolmas—stuffed vine leaves (steamed or baked with variety of fillings)
⬇ Tzatziki—yoghurt cucumber and garlic dip, can be used as dressing
⬇ Plaki—fish broiled in tomato sauce and garlic
⬇ Baba ghanoush—eggplant dip
⬇ Shish kebab—skewered, broiled meat and vegetables
⬇ Gyro—roasted minced lamb with grilled onion, capsicum and tzatziki
⬇ Souvlaki—marinated lamb with lemon, herbs and olive oil

Greek menu

Appetiser/Salad
Greek Salad
Dolmas

Main
Plaki
or
Souvlaki

Dessert
Fresh fruit

Mexican cuisine

Traditional Mexican cuisine is based on corn, beans, chilli, veg-etables and lean meats, and is therefore low in fat. Mexican cuisine served in Australia, the United States and other West-ern countries is prepared with more fat. However, there are some delicious low-fat dishes to enjoy.

Terms meaning more fat

⇧ Crispy
⇧ Chile rellenos—fried cheese parcels
⇧ Chile con queso—cream cheese and chilli
⇧ Chimichangas—fried burritos
⇧ Layered with refried beans
⇧ Mixed with chorizo (Mexican sausage)
⇧ Nachos and cheese
⇧ Served in a crisp tortilla basket
⇧ Sopapillas—Mexican fried bread
⇧ Smothered in cheese sauce
⇧ Guacomole
⇧ Sour cream

Terms meaning less fat

⇩ Asada—grilled
⇩ Mole sauce—chilli-based sauce
⇩ Salsa verde—green chilli sauce
⇩ Salsa—tomato and chilli-based dips
⇩ Picante—spicy
⇩ Veracruz-style—tomato sauce
⇩ Wrapped in soft tortilla

Nutritious menu choices

Appetisers
- ✓ Jicama with fresh lime juice
- ✓ Salsa with fresh vegetables
- ✓ Steamed vegetables

Soups
- ✓ Black bean soup
- ✓ Gazpacho

Mains
- ✓ Soft tacos
- ✓ Burritos, temales, fajitas
- ✓ Red beans and rice
- ✓ Spanish rice
- ✓ Arroz con pollo—chicken with rice
- ✓ Red snapper Veracruz-style
- ✓ Seafood in green chilli sauce

Desserts
- ✓ Fresh fruit
- ✓ Oranges in syrup
- ✓ Candied lime
- ✓ Papaya sorbet

Mexican menu

Appetiser/Salad

Salsa with fresh vegetables

Soup

Gazpacho

Main

Arroz con Pollo

(Chicken with rice)

Dessert

Oranges in syrup

Chinese cuisine

There are a number of Chinese cuisines, including:

Cantonese—well known for its roasted and grilled meats, steamed
   dishes, stir-fried dishes and mild flavours.
Szechuan and *Hunan*—hot and spicy and generally may be higher
   in fat.
Peking—subtle flavours.
Mandarin—aristocratic cuisine. Menu features the finest selection of dishes from all regions.

The art of choosing from the Chinese menu

Within your fat budget: enjoy	Only on credit: avoid
Soups	
Clear broth, egg drop, hot and sour, chicken and corn	
Appetisers	
Steamed spring rolls, steamed dim sims	Deep-fried spring rolls, won tons, dim sims, crab rangoons, egg omelette
Main dishes	
Braised, roasted, simmered, steamed	Pastry or batter-dipped meats
Stir-fried in less oil (ask for less oil to be used)	Deep-fried (e.g. honey chicken, sweet and sour pork), Peking duck, fried fish

Vegetables

Plain steamed, stir-fried, braised

Fried and deep-fried
vegetables

Rice and noodles

Steamed, boiled plain

Fried rice or noodles

Desserts

Oranges, mandarins

Deep-fried ice-cream

Fortune cookies

Nutritious menu choices

Appetisers/salads

✓ Four seasons Chinese vegetables

✓ Steamed dim sims

✓ Steamed spring rolls

Soups

✓ Chicken and corn soup

✓ Long soup

✓ Short soup

✓ Won ton soup

Mains

✓ Beef chow mein

✓ Beef in black bean sauce

✓ Beef in Mandarin sauce

✓ Chicken chop suey

✓ Curried prawns and steamed rice

✓ Garlic prawns

✓ Lobster with ginger and shallots

✓ Scallops in ginger and shallots

✓ Seafood hotpot

Desserts

✓ Chang fen—stuffed sweet rice rolls

✓ Fresh orange

✓ Fortune cookie

Chinese menu

Appetiser/Salad

Steamed spring rolls

Main

Lobster with ginger and
shallots

Braised vegetables

Steamed rice

Dessert

Chang fen

(Stuffed sweet rice rolls)

Japanese cuisine

Japanese cuisine is naturally low in fat, so there is plenty to choose from.

Terms meaning more fat

⇧ Tempura

⇧ Agemono

⇧ Katsu

Terms meaning less fat

⇩ Mushimono or tamaga-yaki—steamed

⇩ Nikogori—in aspic

⇩ Nimono—simmered

⇩ Sunomono or aemono—vinegared

⇩ Yaki—broiled

⇩ Yakimono—grilled, usually, but can be pan-fried or baked

⇩ Sashimi—sliced raw seafood

⇩ Sushi

Nutritious menu choices

Appetisers/salads

✓ Fish sukiyaki—fish hotpot

✓ Miso

✓ Mizu-taki—chicken pot

✓ Nerimono—steamed fish cakes

✓ Niku—Japanese mixed grill

✔ Shabu shabu—beef in broth

✔ Sakana—seafood mixed grill

✔ Salmon nabe—salmon hotpot

✔ Sashimi and sushi

✔ Seafood sunomono—seafood in vinegar sauce

✔ Stir-fried tofu

✔ Vegetable sunomono—side dishes of vegetables in vinegar

Mains

✔ Fish sukiyaki—fish hotpot

✔ Mizu-taki—chicken pot

✔ Niku—Japanese mixed grill

✔ Sakana—seafood mixed grill

✔ Salmon nabe—salmon hotpot

✔ Shabu shabu – beef in broth

✔ Teriyaki chicken

✔ Yakisana—choice of grilled fish

Desserts

✔ Candied chestnuts

✔ Furutsu anmitsu—jellied fruit

✔ Kudanomo—seasonal fruit

✔ Strawberry jelly and yokan jelly

✔ Sweet red bean soup

Japanese menu
Appetiser/Salad
Mixed sushi
Tofu salad
Main
Niku
(Japanese mixed grill)
Vegetable Sunomono
(Side dishes of vegetables)
Gohan
(Steamed rice)
Dessert
Furutsu Anmitsu
(Jellied fruit)

Understanding Japanese culinary terms

Daikon—giant radish

Ito kezuri—dried bonito

Kanten—seaweed aspic

Makunochi—dinner/lunch boxes

Mirin—sweet cooking sake
Miso—fermented bean soup
Mitsumane—jellied fruit
Nori—wraparound sushi
Suimono—clear soup
Togarashi—hot red chilli pepper
Umeboshi—pickled apricots
Yokan—red bean
Zenzai—sweet red bean soup

Korean

Korean cuisine offers a wide variety of wonderfully spiced low-fat dishes.

Nutritious menu choices

Appetisers/salads

- Hobakmuchim—courgettes with beef
- Kakdooki—white radish pickle
- Ke-tchim—steamed crab
- Kujolpan—nine-section appetiser
- Kulhoe—oysters
- Maeuctana—Korean fish stew
- Ojhingubokum—stir-fried squid with chillies and vegetables
- Paejusanjok—grilled scallop kebabs
- Posot—baked mushrooms
- Posotbokkum—mushrooms with chicken and vegetables
- Saengsongui—grilled fish
- Yukhoe—Korean steak tartare
- Khajinamul—aubergine salad
- Kimchi—cabbage pickle
- Kongnamul—beansprout salad
- Muusaengchae—white radish salad
- Mou Sangchae—carrot and white radish salad
- Namul—lotus root salad
- Oinamul—cucumber salad
- Shigumchinamul—spinach salad
- Yachaejorim—soy-glazed pumpkin

Soups

- Kakguk—white radish soup

✓ Manduguk—dumpling soup

✓ Miyoguk—seaweed soup

✓ Mou-kuk—beef soup

✓ Naengmyon—cold buckwheat soup

✓ Shikumchiguk—spinach soup

✓ Takguk—chicken soup with clams and spinach

Mains

✓ Chongol—beef and vegetable hotpot

✓ Pulgogi—grilled beef (ask for sirloin)

✓ Soegogochubokkum—stir-fried beef with garlic and chilli

✓ Takkooe—marinated chicken breast

✓ Tak—stir-fried chicken

✓ Taksanjok—chicken and spring onion kebabs

✓ Twoenjangchigae—beef, bean curd and vegetable hotpot

Rice and noodles

✓ Chapchae—cellophane noodles with lean beef and vegetables

✓ Kijangbap—rice with millet

✓ Kuksu—cold noodles with vegetables

✓ Pibimbap—rice with mixed vegetables

✓ Poribap—rice with barley

✓ Posotbap—rice with mushrooms and beef

✓ Tofu—poached bean curd

Desserts

✓ Fresh fruit

Korean menu

Appetiser/Salad

Manduguk

(Dumpling soup)

Ke-tchim

(Steamed crab)

Mou Sangchae

(Carrot and white radish
salad)

Main

Soegogochubokkum

(Stir fried beef with garlic
and chilli)

Steamed rice

Dessert

Fruit

Thai cuisine

Thai cuisine, with its wonderful aromatic dishes full of flavour and freshness, is probably one of the most loved cuisines around the world.

Nutritious menu choices

Appetisers/salads
- ✔ Chive Nung—chive dumplings
- ✔ Dom Yom Hoy Mang Poo—hot and sour mussels
- ✔ Kanom Jeeb—steamed won tons
- ✔ Lab Tohoo—spicy tofu
- ✔ Lob Gai—spicy ground chicken
- ✔ Look Chin Gai—chicken balls
- ✔ Pad Tohoo Gob Tua Ngog—stir-fried tofu and bean sprouts
- ✔ Paw Pia Sod—steamed spring rolls
- ✔ Pla Goong—spicy shrimp
- ✔ Saku Sai Mu—tapioca with stuffing
- ✔ Yahng Moo—barbecued pork
- ✔ Som Tam—green papaya salad
- ✔ Yam Goong Haeng—dried shrimp salad
- ✔ Yum Nue—beef salad
- ✔ Yam Talae—seafood salad
- ✔ Yum Yai—Thai salad
- ✔ Yum Wun Sen—transparent noodle salad

Soups
- ✔ Ba Mee Nam Muu—pork and noodle soup
- ✔ Gaeng Leuang—yellow curry soup
- ✔ Gaeng Liang—vegetable and prawn soup

Thai menu

Appetisers/Salad

Paw Pia Sod

(Steamed spring rolls)

Soup

Gaeng Liang

(Vegetable and prawn soup)

Main

Gai Pad King (chicken

with ginger)

Pad Tua Song Yang

(Stir-fried green beans and

sprouts)

Steamed rice

Dessert

Seasonal fresh fruit

✓ Tom Yam Gai—spicy chicken soup

✓ Tom Yam Goong—spicy prawn soup

Mains

✓ Bla Nuang—ginger steamed fish

✓ Gai Pad King—chicken with ginger

✓ Gai Pad Mamuang Him Ma Pan—chicken and cashews

✓ Kao Moo Daeng—rice and red pork

✓ Kao Mun Gai—rice and chicken

✓ Moo Wan—sweet pork

✓ Nue Nam Tok—grilled beef with Thai seasoning

✓ Pla Muk Pad Prik Yuok—squid with capsicum

✓ Pla Prio Wan—sweet and sour fish

✓ Pla Sam Rot—three-flavoured fish

✓ Rad Na Gai—noodles with chicken and broccoli

✓ Sen Mee Pad Gai—rice vermicelli with chicken

Vegetable dishes

✓ Pad Galumblee—stir-fried cabbage

✓ Pad Tua Song Yang—fried green beans and sprouts

Desserts

Unfortunately, most Thai desserts are based on coconut, which is rich in saturated fat. Here are a couple that are not:

✓ Tropical fresh fruit

✓ Wun Nam Chuam—agar with syrup

Malaysian cuisine

Malaysian cuisine is a melting pot of Arabic, Indian, Indonesian and Chinese influences. The dominating flavours of Malaysian cuisine are coconut, satay, chilli and curries. Seafood is very popular, as is rice.

Nutritious menu choices

Appetisers/salads

✓ Malay mixed vegetables

✓ Pickled vegetables

✓ Satay with sweet sauce

✓ Steamed rice cakes served with sambal (dipping sauce)

Soups

✓ Hokkien Mee—noodle soup

✓ Tom Yam Kung—prawn soup

Mains

✓ Cabai Meruk Ayam—chicken cooked with red chilli

✓ Daging Masak Sayur—tender meat with vegetables

✓ Grilled whole fish (e.g. red snapper in spicy soy sauce)

✓ Itih Rempah—spicy duck (traditionally skinned)

✓ Memorak Daging Lembu—beef braised in soy sauce

✓ Otak Otak—fish steamed in banana leaves

✓ Satang Masak Hitam—squid in dark sauce

✓ Tamarind beef or chicken

Desserts

✓ Almond jelly

✓ Fresh tropical fruit (e.g. papaya, pineapple, durian (the 'king of fruits'), white mango)

Malaysian menu

Appetiser/Salad
Steamed rice cakes
with sambal (dipping sauce)

Soup
Manduguk
(Dumpling soup)

Main
Grilled red snapper
in spicy soy sauce
Malay mixed vegetables
Steamed rice

Dessert
Es Campur
(Fruits with flavoured ice
topping)

✅ Lychee pudding
✅ Mango jellies

Understanding Malaysian culinary terms

Mee—egg or yellow noodles
Beekoon—rice noodles
Rempah —low-fat spices ground to a paste
Tamarind—sweet tart-flavoured pod used to flavour chicken and beef
Rendang—coconut milk-based curry
Roti Jala—bread made of coconut and flour mixture

Some like it hot

If you feel up to very hot food, keep the following in mind:

- If the heat gets too much, eat natural yoghurt with or without cucumber (as in a cucumber dip). Yoghurt is truly the fire extinguisher, so have it ready with a hot meal.
- Take sips of cold water in between to cool your mouth.
- End your meal with steamed or boiled rice or bread. It helps to absorb the chilli taste.

Indonesian cuisine

Indonesian cuisine uses fragrant, exotic spices, coconut, peanuts, sweet coconut palm syrup, chilli, garlic, ginger and shallots in many combinations to produce a variety of fragrant dishes. Those based on coconut milk are high in saturated fat. Fortunately, there are many nutritious and flavoursome dishes to choose from.

Terms meaning more fat

⬆ Rendang—coconut milk-based curry

⬆ Sayurs—dishes cooked with vegetables (usually crisp-cooked and in coconut sauce)

Terms meaning less fat

⬇ Asam Pedas—'sour hot' fish or meat cooked in very hot, sour gravy

⬇ Gulai—usually coconut-based curry ⬆ or a sauce made from tamarind or pineapple ⬇

⬇ Longton—rice dumpling

⬇ Padang—very hot and spicy

⬇ Panggang—food roasted over a fire

Nutritious menu choices

Appetisers

✓ Bihun Goreng—stir-fried vermicelli with vegetables

✓ Rujak Buah Buahan—fruit plate

✓ Satay prawns

✓ Soup with prawns and noodles

✓ Acar Bening—cucumber relish

✓ Acar Campur Kuning—variety of relishes

✓ Boiled vegetables and chilli condiments

✓ Botok Tahu—steamed spiced bean curd in banana leaves

Soups—often served as a main course

✓ Baso—meatball soup

✓ Rawon—aromatic beef soup

✓ Sayur Asam—snake bean soup and tamarind

✓ Sayur Menir—spinach and corn soup

✓ Sop Ayam Java—Javanese chicken soup

✓ Soto Daging a la Madura—unique Madura beef and vegetable soup

Mains

✓ Ayam Panggang Bumbu Rujak—grilled chicken in sweet spicy sauce

✓ Ayam Saus Jeruk Nipis—roast chicken with lemon sauce

✓ Brengkes Tongkol—baked tuna in sauce and banana leaves

✓ Cap Cap Spesial—special chop suey

✓ Gado Gado—egg and fresh greens spicy salad

✓ Ikan Panggang Bumbu Rujak—grilled fish and aromatic sauce

✓ Kurmah—veal in aromatic sauce

✓ Pangek Bungkus—fish in banana leaves

✓ Sate Ayam Madura—chicken satay Madura-style

✓ Sate Daging Bumbu Rujak—meat satay with red blazing sauce

✓ Singgang Ayam Padang—grilled chicken Padang-style

✓ Sweet soy sauce pork

✓ Udang Laut Saus Kecap—lobster in soy sauce

Desserts

✓ Buah Buahan Dengan Saus Mangga—tropical fruit salad in mango sauce

✓ Fresh tropical fruits

✓ Pisary Sisu—milk banana

✓ Podeng—fruit with agar agar and vanilla sauce

Indonesian menu

Appetisers/Salad

Satay prawns

Acar Campur Kuning

(Variety of relishes)

Main

Ayam Bali

(Chicken in chilli and saffron)

Steamed rice

Dessert

Podeng

(Fruit with agar agar)

Singaporean cuisine

Singaporean cuisine is a blend of Chinese, Indonesian and Malay cooking. You may wish to refer to each of these cuisines for more ideas.

Nutritious menu choices

Appetisers/salads
- Popiah—Hokkien-style fresh spring rolls
- Rojak—salad with spicy sauce
- Satay Babi
- Spicy Kangkung—leafy green vegetables
- Steamed spring rolls
- Stuffed bean curd in crabmeat sauce
- Vegetarian beehoon

Soup
- Hae Mee—prawn noodle soup

Mains
- Hainanese chicken and rice
- Ikan Pari Panggang—BBQ stingray
- Kway Teow—fresh rice-flour noodles and seafood
- Macchi Tandoori and Raita—marinated baked fish and yoghurt dressing
- Steamed sea bass with sauce
- Tea-smoked sea bass, or steamed sea bass with spicy sauce
- Teochew fish

Dessert
- Fresh tropical fruit

Singaporean menu

Appetiser/Salad
Popiah
(Hokkien-style fresh spring rolls)
Rojak
(Salad with spicy sauce)

Main
Ikan Pari Panggang
(BBQ stingray)

Dessert
Fruit

Aeroplane food

If you fly frequently, you may want to pre-order your meals from the low-fat meal selection. By ordering a low-fat meal you will save a lot of fat grams in your daily 'fat account'. A low-fat meal is likely to contain more vegetables and fruit and so will boost your antioxidant intake. Thus, it meets two of the goals for optimal nutrition: lowered fat intake and increased antioxidant intake. You will also get your specially ordered meal ahead of the other passengers! Major airlines cater for low-fat diets, and most cater for vegetarians. You need to notify the airline of your requirements at least 24 hours in advance.

THE IMPORTANCE OF FLUIDS

Dehydration is common during long international flights. The air-conditioned cabin may give you a false security of being cool and you may not necessarily feel thirsty or sweaty. Therefore, you are less likely to drink fluids. But the recycled air is very dry—it's possible, to lose as much as 1 per cent of body fluids during a two-hour flight. This is enough to make it difficult for your body to cool you efficiently. Drinking alcohol makes things worse, as alcohol increases the loss of fluid from your body.

Dehydration makes jet lag worse. The signs of being dehydrated are a headache and fatigue. Your body needs to adjust to the time change, and dealing with dehydration at the same time makes headaches, queasiness and fatigue more probable.

Hints to protect from dehydration

✔ Drink water, fruit juice or tea at least every second hour.

✔ If drinking alcohol, choose mixed drinks with soda water, fruit juice, diet soft drinks or tonic water. Examples: vodka and orange, scotch and soda, gin and diet tonic.

✖ Avoid straight alcoholic drinks.

✔ Drink a big glass of water or fruit juice as soon as you get to your destination.

Further reading

Bellisle, F. et al. 'Functional food science and behaviour and psychological functions', *British Journal of Nutrition,* 80 Suppl. 1, August 1998, pp. S173–93

Bendich, A. 'Antioxidant vitamins and human immune responses', *Vitamins and Hormones*, vol. 52, 1996, pp. 35–62

Benton, D. 'Symposium on nutrition and cognitive function', *Proceedings of the Nutrition Society,* 51, 1992, pp. 295–302

Christensen, L. and Clare Redig, 'Effects of meal composition on mood', *Behavioral Neuroscience,* vol. 107, no. 2, 1993, pp. 346–53

Constant, J. 'Alcohol, ischemic heart disease, and the French paradox', *Clinical Cardiology,* vol. 20, no. 5, 1997, pp. 420–4

Denke, M.A. 'Cholesterol lowering diets: a review of the evidence', *Archives of Internal Medicine,* vol. 155, 9 January 1995, pp. 17–26

Gutierez, Fuentes J.A. 'What food for the heart', *World Health Forum*, vol. 17, 1996

Haber, B. 'The Mediterranean diet: a view from history', *American Journal of Clinical Nutrition*, no. 66 (suppl.), 1997, pp. 1053S–7S

Harbige, L.S. 'Nutrition and immunity with emphasis on infection and autoimmune disease', *Nutrition and Health*, vol. 10, 1996, pp. 285–312

Harris, W.S. 'n-3 fatty acids and serum lipoproteins: human studies', *American Journal of Clinical Nutrition*, vol. 65 (suppl.), 1997, pp. 1645S–54S

Hathcock, J.N. 'Vitamins and minerals: efficacy and safety', *American Journal of Clinical Nutrition*, vol. 66, 1997, pp. 427–37

Hoffman, R.M. and Garewel, H. S. 'Antioxidants and the prevention of coronary heart disease', *Archives of Internal Medicine*, vol. 155, 13 February 1995, pp. 241–6

Kanarek, R. 'Psychological effects of snacks and altered meal frequency', *British Journal of Nutrition*, April 77 Suppl 1 pp. S105–18

McCann, B., Harnick, G. R. and Knopp R. H. 'Changes in plasma lipids and dietary intake accompanying shifts in perceived workload and stress', *Psychosomatic Medicine*, vol. 52, 1990, pp. 97–108

Meyers, D.G., Maloney P. A. and Weeks D. 'Safety of antioxidant vitamins', *Archives of Internal Medicine*, vol. 156, 13 May 1996, pp. 925–35

Mori, T.A., Vanolongen K., Beilin I.J., Burke V., Morris J., Ritchie J. 'Effects of varying dietary fat, fish, and fish oils on blood lipids in a randomised controlled trial in men at risk of heart disease', *American Journal of Clinical Nutrition*, vol. 59, 1994, pp. 1060–8

Smith, A., Kendrick A. and Maben A. 'Use and effects of foods and drinks in relation to daily rhythms of mood and cognitive performance', *Proceedings of the Nutrition Society*, vol. 51, 1992, pp. 325–33

Vinson, J.A. 'Flavonoids in foods as in vitro and in vivo antioxidants', *Advances in Experimental Medical Biology*, vol. 439, 1998, pp. 151–64

Wahlqvist, M.L., Metzger E. D. and Stellor C. 'Food variety as nutritional therapy', *Current Therapeutics*, March, 1997

Wolfe, B. 'The effects of dieting on plasma tryptophan concentration and food intake in healthy women', *Physiology and Behavior*, vol. 61, no. 4, 1997, pp. 537–41

Conversions

1 cup	= 250 ml		1 teaspoon	= 5 ml
¼ cup	= 60 ml		½ teaspoon	= 2.5 ml
⅓ cup	= 80 ml		1 tablespoon	= 20 ml
½ cup	= 125 ml			

Mass (weight)

Metric	Imperial	Metric	Imperial
15 g	½ oz	315 g	10 oz
30 g	1 oz	345 g	11 oz
60 g	2 oz	375 g	12 oz (¾ lb)
90 g	3 oz	410 g	13 oz
120 g	4 oz (¼ lb)	440 g	14 oz
155 g	5 oz	470 g	15 oz
185 g	6 oz	500 g (0.5 kg)	16 oz (1 lb)
220 g	7 oz	750 g	24 oz (1½ lb)
250 g	8 oz (½ lb)	1000 g (1 kg)	32 oz (2 lb)
280 g	9 oz		

Liquids

Metric	Cup	Imperial
30 ml		1 fl oz
60 ml	¼ cup	2 fl oz
90 ml		3 fl oz
120 ml	½ cup	4 fl oz
150 ml		5 fl oz (¼ pint)
200 ml	1 cup	6 fl oz
250 ml	1 cup	8 fl oz
300 ml	1¼ cups	10 fl oz (½ pint)
375 ml	1½ cups	12 fl oz
425 ml	1¾ cups	14 fl oz
475 ml		15 fl oz
500 ml	2 cups	16 fl oz
600 ml	2½ cups	20 fl oz (1 pint)

Index

12345 food and nutrition plan 26

absorption 16–8
  calcium 17
  iron 16–17
  zinc 17–18
acetylcholine 121, 134
activity level 46
adipose tissue 42, 60
adrenalin 111, 121
adrenocorticotrophic hormone
    (ACTH) 112
aerobic power 55
aeroplane food 168–9
  fluids 168–9
  low fat diets 168
  vegetarianism 168
aging 103
  free radicals and 104
alcohol passim
  intoxication with 117
  kilojoule content 40
  replenishing nutrients after 117
  standard drinks 116–17
allostatic load 113
alpha linolenic acid 5, 86

amino acids
  essential 6
  food sources 6
  function 6
  neurotransmitters and 122
android obesity 63
angina 68
angioplasty 69
anthocyanidins 103, 107
anthocyanins 91
antibiotics 95–6
antioxidants 33, 90–2, 96–107
  aging 103
  assessing intake 100–1
  beta carotene 98
  boosting intake 101–3
  drinks rich in 105–7
  food colour and 102–3
  food sources 90
  fruit content 107
  increased needs for 97
  role in immunity 97–107
  rosemary and 103
  supplements 98, 105
  various compounds 99–100
  vitamin C 98
  vitamin E 98

anxiety 133
  tea and 133
ANZFA 30
apple shape 62
arthritis 33
atherosclerosis 66–7
  inherited predisposition to 66
average energy needs 45–7

basic food groups 27
beta carotene 98, 102
  food sources 102
bioavailability 13–18
  calcium 13–17
  iron 13–17
  vegetarian diet 15
  zinc 13–18
bioflavonoids 100
blood brain barrier 122
body composition 55, 60
body fat 60
  consequences of too little 60
  consequences of too much 60
body weight
  gain 43, 47
  loss 4, 47–8
brain development 122
  fatty acids and 122
brain performance 120–35
  role of nutrition 121–3
breakfast
  nutritious examples 124
  spatial memory 124
  word recall 124

cafestol 92
caffeine 93
  in carbonated beverages 133
  in coffee 133
calcium absorption 17
calculating
  energy needs 45–7
  Maximum Heart Rate (MHR) 57

optimal daily fat intake 78
optimal daily fish oil intake 89
waist to hip ratio 63
carbohydrate
  complex 41
  definition 5
  function 41
  in exercise 53–4
  kilojoule content 40
  simple 41
cardiovascular fitness 54–9
  levels 55–9; beginners 55–6;
    intermediate 56
carnosic acid 103
catechins 103, 107
checkpoints
  antioxidants 97, 100–1
  assessing food variety 26–7
  exercise routine 61–2
  fat in your diet 48–51
  nutrients in your diet 8–9
  risk for heart disease 67
  safe upper levels for supplements
    34
  stress inducing habits 109
Chinese cuisine
  choosing healthy choices 153–4
  nutritious menu choices 154–5
  nutritious menu example 155
cholesterol 70–4
  cut off points for 70–1; in Australia
    70; in Europe 70; in National
    Heart Foundation 70; USA 70
  diet therapy for raised 72–93
  HDL cholesterol 70
  LDL cholesterol 70
  medication to lower 71–2
  saturated fat and 73–4
  tests 70–1
cholesterol plaque 68
choline 134–5
  alcohol and 135
  best food sources 135

boosting intake 135
daily recommendations for, 134
memory and 134
supplementation 134; choline
    bitartrate 135; choline chloride
    135; lecithin 135
chronic fatigue 126
circadian rhythm 125
coconut fat 74
coffee
    caffeine content 133
    cholesterol raising effect 92–3
        dehydrating effect 116
    triglyceride raising effect 93
cognitive function 120–135
    alcohol and 123
    blood sugar levels 122; and
        breakfast 124
    meal composition 123–4
    meal timing 124, 127
    role of carbohydrate 127–30; blood
        sugar levels 128–9; glycaemic
        index 128; nutritious snacks
        129–30
complex carbohydrate 127–9
    snacks rich in 129
    see also carbohydrate
copper 99
coronary artery bypass 69
corticotrophin 112
cortisol 112

dehydration 168
    hints to avoid 169
    while flying 168–9; and alcohol
        168; and jetlag 168
decosahexaenoic acid (DHA) 33, 86
diabetes 131
dietary cholesterol 75–6
    food sources 75
    recommended intake 75
    seafood and 76

dietary fat 5, 48–51, 77–85
    content in foods 82–3
    definition 5
    keeping track of 80–2
    kilojoule content 40
    optimal daily amount 78–9
    recommendations for 77–8
dietary induced thermogenesis 41–2
dieting
    consequences of 118–19
    negative behaviours 142
    serotonin production 118
    tryptophan 118
digestion
    carbohydrate 41
    fats 41
    protein 41
diterpenes 92–3
dopamine 123

eating out 141–67
    enjoyment and 141–2
    nutritious meal selection 143–67;
        international cuisines 148–67
    on a 'diet' 142
    positive approach to 142–3
eicosapentaenoic acid (EPA) 33, 86
energy passim
    balance 42–3; negative 43; positive
        43
    body storage sites 42
    content of 40; alcohol 40;
        carbohydrate 40; fats 40;
        protein 40
    food composition 40
    needs 43–7; calculating individual
        45–7
essential amino acids 6
essential fats 85–90
    boosting intake 90
    classification 85
exercise 53–62
    assessing your routine 61–2

benefits of 54
carbohydrate and 53–4
commencing 57
diary 58
flexibility and 59
fuel of choice 53–4
metabolic rate 59
muscular strength and 59
staying in shape and 59

fats *passim*
assessing your intake 48–51
individual fat account 80–2
suggestions to lower intake 51–3
see also dietary fat
fibre
definition 6
free radicals and 105
fight or flight response 111
adrenalin and 111
fish oils 86
blood clots and 86–7
content in fish 89
daily requirements 89
DHA 86
EPA 86
in cold water fish 86–8
triglycerides and 87
fitness 39–64
flavanones 103, 107
flavones 103
flavonols 103, 107
flexibility 55, 59
fluid 6
food groups 22–3, 26–7
food serves
examples of 27
food variety 20–7
assessing 21–2
food colour and 23–4
food diary to assess 21–2
food groups 22–3, 26–7
food serves 27

models 24–6
score 20–1
free radicals
aging and 104
causes 96
DNA damage 104
foods preventing 104–5
foods promoting 104
high fibre foods and 105
overeating and 43
French Paradox 91

glucose 5
glycaemic index 128
blood glucose levels and 131
food selection based on 132
glycogen 42, 53
exercise and 53
Greek cuisine
identifying fatty choices 150
identifying low fat choices 150
nutritious menu example 150
gynecoid obesity 63

healthy weight range 60–1
chart 61
heart attack 69
heart disease 33, 65–93
blood cholesterol and 69–72
development of 68–9
diet and 72–93
risk factors for 67
surgical treatment in 69
vitamin E supplementation 33

immune system 95–6
antioxidants and 96
free radicals and 96
nutrient deficiencies 95–6
nutrition and 95–107
trace elements 99
indole alkaloids 100
indoles 100

Indonesian cuisine
  identifying fatty choices 165
  identifying low fat choices 165
  nutritious menu choices 165–6
  nutritious menu example 166
iron 16–7, 99
  absorption 16–7
irregular meals 128
  blood sugar level and 128
isoflavones 103
Italian cuisine
  identifying fatty choices 148
  identifying low fat choices 148–9
  selecting pizza toppings 149
  nutritious menu example 149

Japanese cuisine
  culinary terms 157–8
  identifying fatty choices 156
  identifying low fat choices 156
  nutritious menu choices 156–7
  nutritious menu example 157

kahwed 92
kilojoule *passim*
  content of alcohol 41;
      carbohydrate 41; fats 41;
      protein 41
  counting 41
Korean cuisine
  nutritious menu choices 159–60
  nutritious menu example 160

lecithin 135
limonoids 100
linoleic acid 5
low fat food selection 84–5
lunch 126
  nutritious choices 126

macronutrients 5–6
  carbohydrates 5
  fats 5

fibre 6
fluid 6
proteins 6
Malaysian cuisine
  culinary terms 164
  hints for eating hot food 164
  nutritious menu choices 163–4
  nutritious menu example 164
manganese 99
Maximal Heart Rate (MHR) 57
maximal oxygen consumption 55
memory 134
menu selections
  Chinese cuisine 153–5
  Greek cuisine 150
  Indonesian cuisine 165–6
  Italian cuisine 148–9
  Japanese cuisine 156–8
  Korean cuisine 159–60
  Malaysian cuisine 163–4
  Mexican cuisine 151–2
  Singaporean cuisine 167
  Thai cuisine 161–2
metabolic rate 44
Mexican cuisine
  identifying fatty choices 151
  identifying low fat choices 151
  nutritious menu choices 152
  nutritious menu example 152
micronutrients
  minerals 7; avoiding losses 12–13;
      best food sources 12–13;
      spotting deficiencies 9
  function 7
  organic 7
  vitamins 7; avoiding losses 10–12;
      best food sources 10–12;
      spotting deficiencies 8
minerals 7, 9, 12–13
  best food sources 12–13
monotrenes 100

mood 123–4, 127–8
  meal composition and 123–4
muscular strength 54, 59

neurons 121
neurotransmitters 121–3
norepinephrine 123
nutrient *passim*
  deficiencies; assessing 8–9;
      correcting 30–2
nutrition *passim*
  food diary to assess 138
  negative effects of dieting 138
  setting personal aims 137
  simple strategies for improvement
      137–9
nutritional supplements 30–5
  alcohol 31
  antioxidant 33
  contraceptive pill 31
  examples of greater need for 31
  preventing deficiencics 30–2
  safe upper levels of intake 34
  safety measures 30, 33–5
  smoking 31
  vegetarianism 31
  use in chronic conditions 33;
      arthritis 33; heart disease 33;
      osteoporosis 33
  w-3 fatty acids 33
nutritious menu selections
  general guide to healthy choices
      143–6; appetisers 145; breads
      146; desserts 146; meat dishes
      146; rice and pasta 146; sauces
      146–7; soups 145; terms
      meaning less fat 144; terms
      meaning more fat 143;
      vegetables 146
  international cuisines 148–67;
      Chinese 153–5; Greek 150;
      Indonesian 165–6; Italian
      148–9; Japanese 156–8; Korean

159–60; Malaysian 163–4;
      Mexican 151–2; Singaporean
      167; Thai 161–2

omega 3 fatty acids
  arthritis 33
  see also w-3 fatty acids
osteoporosis 33
overeating
  ageing and 43
  free radicals and 43

pear shape 62
physical activity 46
  estimating level of 46
physical fitness 54
plant sterols 75–6
  carotenoid absorption and 76
  LDL cholesterol and 76
  spreads enriched with 75–6
polyphenols 91–2
post lunch dip 125–6
  avoiding 126
  circadian rhythm 125
  cortisol and 125
  energy levels during 125
proteins 5
  function 41
  kilojoule content 40
psychological stress 110

reactive hypoglycaemia 130–1
  glycaemic index and 131
  insulin sensitivity and 130
Recommended Dietary Intakes (RDI)
      31–2
  Australia 32
  UK 32
  USA 32
rosemary 103

saturated fat 73–4
  coconut fat and 74

food sources 73
  hints to reduce intake 74
  reading ingredient lists for 74
seafood
  cholesterol and 76–7
selenium 99
serotonin 118, 122, 133
  sleep and 133
Singaporean cuisine
  nutritious menu choices 167
  nutritious menu example 167
sleep problems 132–4
  amino acids and 133
  caffeine and 132
  helpful strategies 134
stress
  adaptations 112
  alcohol and 116–17
  caffeine and 115–16
  counteracting with diet 113–15
  eating habits and 109
  heart rate 113
  hormones 112
  nutrition and 108–19
  physiological effects 113; blood
    lipid levels 113; blood pressure
    and 113; blood sugar levels
    113
supplements 30–5
  see also nutritional supplements
synapse 121

Thai cuisine
  nutritious menu choices 161–2
  nutritious menu example 162
Therapeutic Goods Administration 30

trans fatty acids 74–5
triglycerides 77
tryptophan 6, 118, 122, 133
  serotonin and 122
  sleep and 133
tyrosine 123

viral infections 99
  nutrition and 99
vitamin C 98, 102
  best food sources 102
vitamin E 98–9, 102
  best food sources 102
vitamin P 100
vitamins 7–8, 10–12
  best food sources 10–12
VO_{2max} 55

waist to hip ratio 62–4
  android obesity and 62
  calculating individual 63
  gynecoid obesity and 62
  risk of chronic disease and 62–4
weight loss 4
  golden rules for 47–8
wine 91–2
  antioxidant properties 91
  heart disease and 91–2; optimal
    amounts 92
  polyphenol content 92
w-3 fatty acids 33, 85, 86
  in fish 86–90
w-6 fatty acids 85, 90

zinc absorption 99